Optometric Instrumentation

Optometric Instrumentation

David B. Henson, MSc, PhD, FAAO
Department of Optometry, University of Wales Institute of Science and Technology, Cardiff, Wales

Butterworths
London   Boston   Durban   Singapore   Sydney   Toronto   Wellington

First published 1983

© **Butterworth & Co. (Publishers) Ltd 1983**

British Library Cataloguing in Publication Data

Henson, David B.
  Optometric instrumentation.
  1. Vision–Testing   2. Eye, Instruments
  and apparatus for
  I. Title
  612′.84   RE75

  ISBN 0-407-00241-3

Photoset by Butterworths Litho Preparation Department
Printed and Bound in Great Britain by Page Bros., Norwich, Norfolk

Foreword

The use of instruments in modern optometric practice forms an essential part of the examination of the eye and is an area which has not ceased to evolve. Yet, until now, no one has described all the ophthalmic instruments in one book. This is somewhat surprising when one thinks that many of the instruments which are part of our daily routine were first developed in the nineteenth century.

The discovery of the ophthalmometer by Ramsden in 1795 and its modern version by Helmholtz in 1856 and Javal and Schiotz in 1881 made it possible to measure the curvature of the cornea. The introduction of the ophthalmoscope by Helmholtz in 1851 made possible the examination of the fundus of the living eye, thereby enabling the health of the retina and even of the individual to be monitored. The retinoscope, which Cuignet developed in 1873, started the era of objective examination that has blossomed in the last few years with the appearance of the auto-refractometers. The slit lamp which Gullstrand presented in 1911 to provide a macroscopic view of the anterior segment of the eye found an additional role in the practice of contact lenses. The tonometer, which Maklakov developed in 1885, has been followed by a host of sophisticated instruments enabling us to assess the intraocular pressure. The development of visual field apparatus has been most spectacular and involves more computer utilization than ever before. All these instruments and many others used for various purposes are described in this book.

Dr. Henson has not only covered routine practical equipment, but also many new instruments which are not likely to have found their way, as yet, into practice, but are nonetheless of interest to the practitioner, e.g. the auto-refractometers, the objective acuity devices, the ophthalmic cameras, etc. In fact, some of the new instruments are not mentioned in any other text but this one.

Not content with just a description of the instruments, Dr. Henson has himself drawn numerous diagrams which are not only original and simple to understand, but are also attractive. For most of the equipment, Dr. Henson has cited the relevant studies in which the instrument has been evaluated.

This text is not merely an academic treatise for students, but is also a practical guide in as much as the reader is given a good idea as to the clinical importance of many of the instruments described. It is also very well referenced.

Very helpful to the reader is the fact that Dr. Henson introduces many chapters with a discussion of the theoretical aspects. For example, in the chapter on field equipment there is a description of the type of field defect commonly found in optometric practice and a discussion of the kinetic and static technique of examination. Dr. Henson also touches upon the well known discrepancy found between the results of subjective and retinoscopic examinations, and he presents the latest views on the subject. And the chapter on tonometers even includes a treatment of the basic statistics necessary for the comprehension of studies evaluating the instrument.

This book is a welcome and timely addition to the spectrum of books forming the discipline of optometry. It represents the first of its kind and will prove to be an invaluable tool to the modern practitioner.

Michel Millodot, PhD, OD
Laboratory of Experimental Optometry
UWIST, Cardiff

Contents

1

Ophthalmoscopes

Ophthalmoscopes are used to examine the media and fundus of the eye. The technique of ophthalmoscopy is of such immense value to the medical profession that the majority of textbooks on ophthalmology include large sections on both how to correctly use an ophthalmoscope and how to differentially diagnose the many ocular and systemic conditions that give rise to changes in the media and fundus. Within this chapter I describe the optical systems incorporated in many of the currently produced ophthalmoscopes and mention how certain instrument parameters affect the quality of the fundal image. For a description of how to correctly use an ophthalmoscope and how to diagnose specific conditions from the fundal image, the reader is referred to Michaelson (1980) and Duane (1981).

Instrumentally, ophthalmoscopes can be divided into two groups – direct and indirect. With a direct ophthalmoscope, the practitioner views the retina itself, while with an indirect instrument he views an image of the retina formed by the ophthalmoscope lens. Direct ophthalmoscopes are optically fairly simple. They are invariably hand-held instruments and comprise little more than a bulb, a lens, a reflector and a focusing system. Indirect ophthalmoscopes are much more variable, both in their size and complexity. While some are hand-held instruments which can be used with a natural pupil, others are stand mounted and rely upon the instillation of a mydriatic in order to give a clear view of the fundus.

The angular field of view of direct ophthalmoscopes is considerably less than that of indirect ones. Typically, direct ophthalmoscopes are reported as having a 10–12 degree field of view (the actual extent depends upon several parameters such as the distance of the practitioner from the patient), while indirect ophthalmoscopes can have fields of view that extend up to 60 degrees.

The magnification with which the fundus is viewed also varies with the type of ophthalmoscope. Direct ophthalmoscopes have a magnification of approximately ×15, while indirect ones can have magnifications as low as ×2–3. The upper limit of the magnification with indirect ophthalmoscopes is dependent upon the instrument design, but can be as high as ×40 (Emsley, 1963).

In general, the functional differences between direct and indirect ophthalmoscopes are that with a direct ophthalmoscope the practitioner can see a small part of the fundus under a high magnification, while with an indirect ophthalmoscope a much larger area of the fundus is seen under a much lower magnification. Which of the two systems is best for optometry is a difficult question to answer. Certainly it is true to say that the majority of optometrists currently use direct ophthalmoscopes. This preference can, however, be ascribed to the high costs of indirect ophthalmoscopes and, until recently, to the absence of any compact, hand-held indirect ophthalmoscopes that do not require the use of a mydriatic in order to view the fundus.

A few years ago, American Optical started to produce a hand-held indirect ophthalmoscope which does not require a dilated pupil. This instrument has made it possible for optometrists to routinely use an indirect ophthalmoscope. Several practitioners now advocate the routine use of both indirect and direct instruments. The larger field of view of the indirect instrument makes it ideal for the initial examination, while the high magnification of the direct instrument makes it ideal for the more detailed examination of specific regions of the fundus.

Direct ophthalmoscopes

Optically, these instruments are composed of two parts, an illuminating system and a viewing system. The illuminating system is composed of a tungsten bulb, a condenser system, a lens and a reflector (*see Figure 1.1*). The bulb is usually pre-centred to ensure precise location of the filament's image upon the surface of the reflector. In some instruments, the bulb may be filled with halogen gas which enables the filament to be run at higher temperatures with a consequent increase in light output. The type of reflector used varies from instrument to instrument; some use a small metallic plate, while others use a prism or a mirror.

A range of aperture stops and filters is normally placed between the condensing lens and the projection lens. The apertures allow the practitioner to reduce the size of the illuminated patch upon the retina, a facility which is especially important in the examination of the macula (*see* pp. 5 and 7 for a further description of the effects of aperture stops).

Some of the earlier ophthalmoscopes allowed the practitioner to insert a green filter in the illumination system. This filter, which is sometimes called a red-free filter due to its ability to remove the long wavelength light from the illuminating beam, had two effects upon the fundal appearance. First, it increased the contrast between the retinal vessels and the background and, second, it allowed the practitioner to differentiate between retinal and choroidal lesions; the retinal lesions appeared black, while the choroidal ones appeared grey. This differentation is due to the scattering of short wavelength light by the retinal tissues. These changes in the appearance of the fundus were dependent upon the ophthalmoscope's light source emitting a fairly large amount of short wavelength light. Practically all of today's ophthalmoscopes use tungsten filament bulbs as a light source. While these sources have many advantages over those used in the earlier instruments, one of their disadvantages is that they give out very little short wavelength light. If a red-free filter were to be placed within the illumination system of these instruments, it would absorb the majority of the incident illumination and there would be very little light left to illuminate the patient's fundus. In this situation, any observation of the patient's fundus would be difficult, if not impossible. In order to overcome

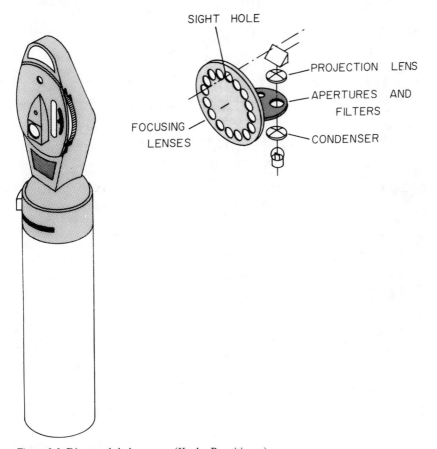

Figure 1.1. Direct ophthalmoscope (Keeler Practitioner)

this problem, manufacturers have compromised in the design of these filters. They now allow fairly large amounts of long wavelength light through. This compromise means that there is only a slight increase in contrast between the retinal vessels and the background and differentiation between retinal and choroidal lesions is correspondingly more difficult.

The viewing system of modern ophthalmoscopes comprises a sight hole and focusing system. The focusing system allows the practitioner to compensate for the combined refractive states of the examiner and the patient and thereby to obtain a clear view of the patient's fundus. The system is usually composed of a rack of lenses of different powers, one of which sits in front of the sight hole. The practitioner focuses upon the patient's fundus by changing the lens in front of the sight hole with a thumbwheel. The majority of ophthalmoscopes have the focusing lenses mounted around the outside of a wheel, as shown in *Figure 1.1*. Others link these together on a chain, as shown in *Figure 1.2*. The latter technique generally allows more lenses to be incorporated in the ophthalmoscope and

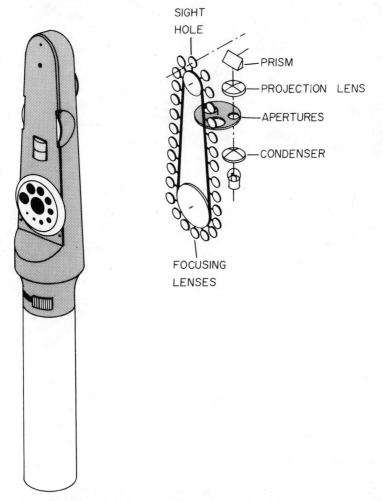

Figure 1.2. Direct ophthalmoscope (Keeler Specialist)

hence offers either a wider focusing range or smaller steps between the powers of the lenses. In addition to the chain or wheel of lenses, most ophthalmoscopes incorporate a high-power positive and a high-power negative lens that, when combined with the chain or wheel of lenses, increase the focusing range.

As mentioned earlier, the focusing lenses are used to compensate for the combined refractive states of the patient and the practitioner. If the practitioner has a high refractive error, then the effective range of the focusing lenses is shifted. For example, an ophthalmoscope that offers a range of lenses that extends from +45 D to −45 D can, with an emmetropic practitioner, be used to view the fundus of any patient whose refractive error falls within the range ±45 D. However, a practitioner who has a refractive error of −10 D will only be able to focus on the fundi of patients whose refractive errors fall within the range of −35 D to +60 D. The ametropic practitioner can compensate for this shift by attaching a contact lens over the sight hole of the ophthalmoscope, whose power equals the refractive error of the practitioner.

The sight hole of the ophthalmoscope, which normally has an aperture of 3 mm, fixes the viewing axis of the instrument slightly to one side of the illumination axis. This arrangement displaces the corneal reflex to one side of the field of view. Without it, the corneal reflex, which is an image of the ophthalmoscope bulb formed by the cornea acting as a convex mirror, would fall in the centre of the field of view and obstruct the practitioner's view of the fundus. The intensity and position of this reflex is dependent upon several parameters, which include:

1. The angle between the illuminating and viewing axes;
2. The distance of the practitioner from the patient;
3. The size of the aperture stop within the illuminating system;
4. The size of the sight hole.

The angle between the illuminating and viewing axes

While an increase of this angle increases the displacement of the reflex, it also reduces the amount of overlap at the retina between the illuminating and viewing systems, i.e. it reduces the amount of illuminated retina visible through the sight hole. For this reason the angle is normally kept fairly small.

The distance of the practitioner from the patient

The physical separation, at the cornea, between the illuminating and viewing paths is dependent upon the distance of the practitioner from the patient. The closer the practitioner is, the greater will be this separation and the further away from the viewing axis will be the corneal reflex. This fact can readily be appreciated in the practitioner's own consulting room. The practitioner merely has to attempt to view the macula at a distance of, say, 10 cm. If he or she now gradually moves towards the patient, the reflex will be seen to gradually move away from the centre of the field of view, which enables the examination of the macula.

The size of the aperture stop within the illumination system

The intensity of the corneal reflex is dependent upon the aperture stop placed within the illumination system. The larger the aperture, the larger will be the cross-sectional area of the illuminating beam at the cornea and

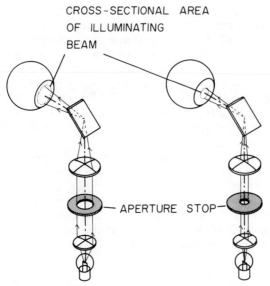

CROSS-SECTIONAL   AREA
OF   ILLUMINATING
BEAM

— APERTURE   STOP—

Figure 1.3. At the cornea the cross-section of the
illuminating beam is dependent upon the aperture stop
within the illuminating system

the greater will be the amount of light reflected back into the viewing
system (*see Figure 1.3*). The importance of this factor appears not to have
been realized by certain manufacturers who fail to provide a stop small
enough to allow the macula to be easily examined.

The size of the sight hole

The corneal reflex is formed approximately 4–5 mm behind the cornea. Its
image, as seen by the practitioner, will be considerably out of focus. The
size of this blurred image will be dependent upon the sight-hole diameter.
As the sight hole is decreased, so too is the size of the blurred image of the
corneal reflex. Reducing the size of the sight hole, however, also reduces
the amount of light for observation. The sight hole of modern ophthalmoscopes is therefore usually kept at about 3–4 mm.

An alternative technique of reducing or, in this case, removing the
corneal reflex is by cross-polarizing the illuminating and viewing systems.
Because the specular reflection from the cornea retains any polarization
while the diffuse reflection from the fundus does not, the effect of
cross-polarizing the illuminating and viewing systems is to selectively
remove the corneal reflex. The disadvantages of this technique, which can
be found in the Keeler Pantoscope, are that, first, a large amount of the
light is lost when it passes through the polarizer and analyzer and, second,
the vessel reflexes, which are specular in origin, are also lost. Many
practitioners feel that these reflexes are valuable for they allow the
practitioner to assess the state of the retinal vessels.

Coincidence of the field of view and field of illumination

In an ideal situation, the field of illumination of an ophthalmoscope should be made to equal the field of view. Increasing the field of illumination beyond the field of view only results in an unnecessary amount of light being shone into the eye. This additional light may, in fact, make examination of the fundus more difficult by further reducing the size of the pupil and thereby reducing the field of view. In addition to this, the larger field of illumination results in a brighter corneal reflex which also makes examination of the fundus more difficult.

The angular field of view with a typical modern ophthalmoscope and a patient with a 3 mm pupil is about 12 degrees. The aperture stop within the viewing system should, therefore, be made to give a field of illumination equal to this value. As it is quite feasible that the ophthalmoscope will occasionally be used to view the fundi of patients with dilated pupils where the field of view will be closer to 20 degrees (6 mm pupil), it is obviously advisable to have a second, larger aperture stop that would increase the field of illumination to about 20 degrees. As mentioned earlier, it is also desirable to have a small aperture stop for viewing the macula. Ideally, direct ophthalmoscopes should contain, therefore, at least three aperture stops: a small one for viewing the macula; an intermediate one for viewing the fundus through normal pupils; and a large one for viewing the fundus through dilated pupils. Unfortunately, many current ophthalmoscopes have only two aperture stops; they leave out either the small or intermediate stops.

The distance of the focusing lens from the cornea in most direct ophthalmoscopes is about 2–3 cm. In cases of high myopia, this relatively large distance results in a considerable degree of fundus magnification which can, in certain cases, be so great that it makes it difficult for the optometrist to examine the fundus. A means of overcoming this problem, advocated by several practitioners, is for the patient to wear his own spectacle correction. Because spectacle corrections are normally placed much closer to the cornea than the focusing lenses of the ophthalmoscope, the amount of magnification is reduced.

Indirect ophthalmoscopes

Indirect ophthalmoscopes differ from direct ones in that the practitioner views an image of the fundus rather than the fundus itself. This image is produced by an ophthalmoscope lens which is placed between the practitioner and the patient. Indirect ophthalmoscopes vary immensely in their size and complexity. Some, such as the American Optical monocular indirect ophthalmoscope, are only fractionally larger than many of the direct instruments. Others, such as the Zeiss (Oberkochen) fundus camera, are so large that they have to be mounted on instrument tables.

The most basic type of indirect ophthalmoscope is shown in *Figure 1.4*. The ophthalmoscope lens, the power of which ranges from +13 to +30 D, is hand held in front of the patient's eye. This lens fulfils two functions: first, it images the exit pupil of the illuminating system and entrance pupil of the viewing system in the patient's pupil; second, it images the patient's fundus at a point between the ophthalmoscope lens and the observer.

The position of the fundal image varies with the refractive state of the patient and the power of the ophthalmoscope lens. For an emmetropic patient and a 13 D ophthalmoscope lens, the fundal image is positioned 77 mm in front of the ophthalmoscope lens. If the practitioner were 60 cm from the ophthalmoscope lens, he would need to exert about 2 D of accommodation in order to see clearly the fundal image. If the patient were hyperopic or the practitioner wished to move closer towards the image in order to increase the magnification with which the fundus is viewed, then further accommodation would have to be exerted. As this is not always possible (e.g. a presbyopic practitioner), indirect ophthalmoscopes of the type shown in *Figure 1.4* invariably incorporate a set of focusing lenses which can be placed in front of the sight hole.

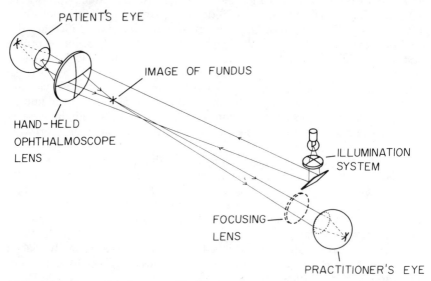

Figure 1.4. Indirect ophthalmoscope. The illumination system is often attached to a head band worn by the practitioner

Ophthalmoscope lenses of higher power decrease the magnification and, for a given diameter of lens, increase the field of view. Because of the difficulties encountered in making good quality, high-power lenses of large aperture, lenses of higher power usually have a smaller diameter and, therefore, do not always give a significantly larger field of view.

The majority of the ophthalmoscope lenses are made with aspheric surfaces in order to reduce their aberrations and increase the quality of the fundal image. The more convex surface of these lenses should face the practitioner.

Since the light source shines through the ophthalmoscope lens, an additional pair of reflexes occurs – one reflex from the front surface of the lens and one from the back. In order to keep the strength of these reflexes to a minimum, the ophthalmoscope lens is usually coated with an anti-reflecting material. Any residual reflection can be displaced from the field of view by tilting the ophthalmoscope lens with respect to the illuminating and viewing axes.

The major advantage of indirect ophthalmoscopy is the relatively large field of view. Its exact angular size is dependent upon the position and aperture of the ophthalmoscope lens. In the simple type of indirect ophthalmoscope shown in *Figure 1.4*, where the lens is typically 16 D with an effective aperture of about 40 mm, the field of view would be approximately 32 degrees. In some of the more elaborate instruments, this has been increased to about 45 degrees by increasing the effective aperture of the ophthalmoscope lens.

Another advantage of indirect ophthalmoscopy is that, with careful design, it is possible to completely remove the corneal reflex from the field of view. Gullstrand was one of the first people to produce a reflex-free ophthalmoscope. He achieved this by separating the illuminating and viewing paths as they passed through the cornea and the lens. When the paths are separated in this way the reflected light from the corneal surface does not enter the viewing system – i.e. it is reflex free. Gullstrand's original design was rather complicated and expensive to produce, and was modified by Henker in 1922. It is the Gullstrand ophthalmoscope as simplified by Henker that forms the basis of most modern indirect ophthalmoscopes (*see Figures 1.5* and *1.6*).

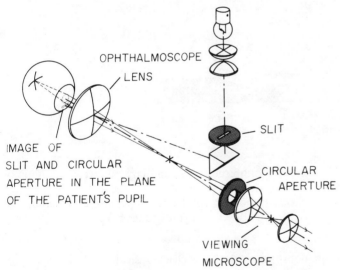

OPHTHALMOSCOPE

LENS

SLIT

IMAGE OF
SLIT AND CIRCULAR
APERTURE IN THE PLANE
OF THE PATIENT'S PUPIL

CIRCULAR
APERTURE

VIEWING
MICROSCOPE

Figure 1.5. The simplified Gullstrand reflex-free indirect ophthalmoscope

Gullstrand's simplified ophthalmoscope passes light into the eye through a narrow slit that is imaged in the plane of the patient's pupil. Observation of the fundus is made through a circular aperture, also imaged in the plane of the patient's pupil. The images of the illumination system's exit pupil (the slit) and the viewing system's entrance pupil (the circular aperture) are separated in the plane of the patient's pupil, as shown in *Figure 1.5*. The entrance pupil of the viewing system is imaged at the centre of the pupil in order to keep the quality of the fundal image as good as possible.

The magnification of an emmetropic patient's fundus with a Gullstrand type of ophthalmoscope is equal to

$$\frac{F}{F_o} \times B$$

where F equal the power of the eye being examined, F_o the power of the ophthalmoscope lens, and B the magnification of the secondary optics. The magnification of the secondary optics can be made to equal almost any value. With very high magnifications there is a reduction in the field of

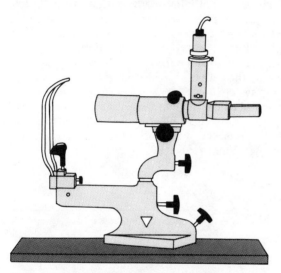

Figure 1.6. The simplified Gullstrand reflex-free ophthalmoscope as made by Bausch and Lomb

view due to difficulties encountered in making large aperture systems of high magnification.

As practically all modern indirect ophthalmoscopes are based upon the Gullstrand design, I will only describe two of them herein.

Monocular indirect ophthalmoscope (American Optical)

The major difference between this indirect ophthalmoscope and many of the other designs is that it is a hand-held instrument that can be used with a natural pupil. This makes it a practical instrument for the routine examination of patients in an optometric practice. Its optical system (*see Figure 1.7*) is based upon the Gullstrand instrument. The filament of the light source is imaged in the plane of the patient's pupil beneath the image of the viewing system's entrance pupil. The area of fundus illuminated by the light source is controlled with an iris diaphragm placed within the illumination system. With this diaphragm, the area of retina illuminated can be made to equal that visible through the viewing system.

The diameter of the ophthalmoscope lens in the American Optical instrument is considerably less than that of other indirect systems, with the effect that the field of view is only about 20 degrees compared with 30 or even 45 degrees in other systems. The 20 degree field of view is still, however, considerably greater than that obtained with a direct instrument, which is usually of the order of about 10 degrees.

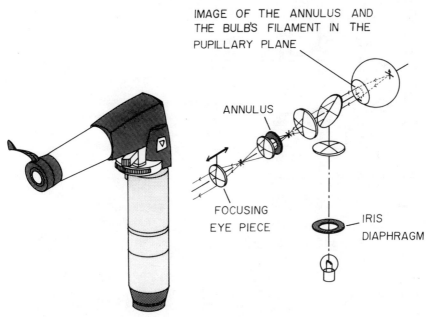

Figure 1.7. Monocular indirect ophthalmoscope (American Optical)

The image of the fundus, formed by the ophthalmoscope lens, is viewed by a compound microscope, the eyepiece of which can be moved back and forth in order to focus the instrument. The use of a compound microscope means that the fundal image is inverted, or rather re-inverted, such that it is now seen erect.

Zeiss (Oberkochen) fundus camera

The Zeiss fundus camera (*see Figure 1.8*) is a stand-mounted indirect ophthalmoscope the optics of which are based upon those of the simplified Gullstrand instrument. It is capable of producing excellent photographs of the fundus, for which it requires a dilated pupil.

The instrument contains two light sources: a tungsten filament for viewing the fundus and focusing the instrument, and a flash source for taking the photograph. The two light sources are optically combined through the semi-reflecting surface shown in *Figure 1.9*.

The light from the two light sources passes through a diaphragm, the adjustment of which controls the size of the illuminated patch upon the patient's retina. This diaphragm is imaged at the surface of a fenestrated

12

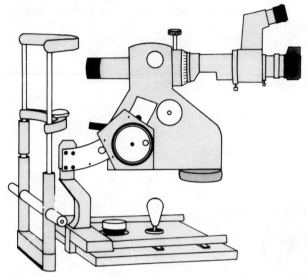

Figure 1.8. Fundus camera (Zeiss (Oberkochen))

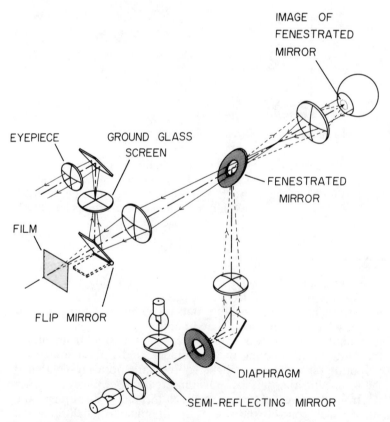

Figure 1.9. Isometric diagram of the optics of the Zeiss (Oberkochen) fundus camera

mirror, which is itself imaged by the ophthalmoscope lens in the plane of
the patient's pupil. These two optical elements confine the illuminating
beam to an annulus the width of which is controlled by the diaphragm.

The ophthalmoscope lens produces an image of the fundus between the
fenestrated mirror and the ophthalmoscope lens. This image is viewed
through the fenestration with a compound microscope. The objective of
this microscope forms an image of the fundus, via flip mirror, upon a
ground glass screen which is placed at the focal point of the viewing
eyepiece. As the photograph is taken, the flip mirror moves out of the path
of the viewing system which enables the image produced by the viewing
microscope's objective to fall upon the photographic film. The ground
glass screen within the viewing system ensures that the image produced at
the film plane will be at least as sharp as that seen through the eyepiece.
Without this screen it would be possible, by having the eyepiece incorrectly
set, to have a clear image through the viewing microscope and when the
mirror is flipped out of the way, a blurred image at the film plane.

The fenestrated mirror, which is imaged by the ophthalmoscope lens in
the plane of the patient's pupil, forms the entrance pupil of the viewing
system. It confines the viewing beam to the central region of the pupil. It
also confines the illuminating beam to an annulus that surrounds the
viewing beam. The illuminating and viewing paths are therefore separated
in the plane of the patient's pupil, thereby making the instrument reflex
free.

The Zeiss fundus camera has a 30 degree field of view and, as mentioned
earlier, is capable of producing excellent photographs of the fundus. While
the instrument is not suitable for the routine examination of the fundus it is
a very good example of how indirect ophthalmoscopes have been developed in order to obtain photographs of the fundus. All fundus cameras
are indirect ophthalmoscopes and, currently, they are all based upon the
principles of Gullstrand's ophthalmoscope.

References

DUANE, T. D. (1981). *Clinical Ophthalmology*. Harper and Row, Philadelphia
EMSLEY, H. H. (1963). *Visual Optics*, Vol. II. Hatton Press, London
MICHAELSON, I. C. (1980). *Textbook of the Fundus of the Eye*. Churchill and Livingstone,
    Edinburgh

2

Retinoscopes

Retinoscopy is a simple, objective means of obtaining the refractive error of an eye. Optically, modern retinoscopes are composed of a single lens, a light source and a mirror. The mirror either has a hole drilled in it or is made to semi-reflect such that the retinoscopist can view the patient's eye along the retinoscope's beam of light (*see Figure 2.1*).

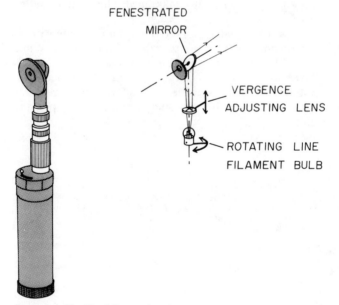

FENESTRATED
MIRROR

VERGENCE
ADJUSTING LENS

ROTATING LINE
FILAMENT BULB

Figure 2.1. The Hamblin streak retinoscope

Before describing retinoscopes in more detail, I will briefly mention the basic principles upon which retinoscopy is based and the different techniques used to find the axis of astigmatic errors. A more detailed description of the technique of retinoscopy can be found in most ophthalmic text books, including Emsley (1963), Bennett and Francis (1964), Borish (1970) and Duke-Elder (1970).

Principles of retinoscopy

In retinoscopy, the observer views a small patch of light formed upon the fundus of the patient's eye. By moving the patch in a given direction and viewing the direction in which it appears to move after being refracted by the patient's eye, the retinoscopist is able to say whether the patient's retina is focused in front of, at or behind his own eye. The refractive error is measured by placing lenses in front of the patient's eye until the patient's retina is focused at the retinoscopist's eye.

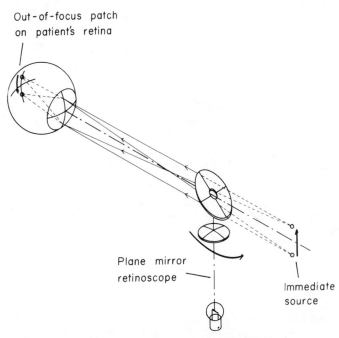

Figure 2.2. The formation of a blurred patch of light upon the patient's retina. The arrows indicate that as the retinoscope's mirror is tilted down so the patch of light on the patient's retina also moves down

Figure 2.2 shows how a plane mirror retinoscope (the type most commonly used today) forms an out-of-focus patch of light upon the patient's fundus. It also shows that when the mirror is tilted down this patch of light also moves down. While the actual size of the patch varies with different degrees of ametropia, the direction of movement does not.

This patch of light now becomes the object in the following two cases. The first (*Figure 2.3*) is for a hyperope of less than 1.50 D, and the second (*Figure 2.4*) for a myope. The point to notice from these two figures is that there is an aerial image of the retinal patch formed either behind or in front of the retinoscopist's eye and that this aerial image moves in the opposite direction to the movement of the retinal patch. Thus, if the retinal patch moves down the aerial image moves up.

Figures 2.5 and *2.6* show how this aerial image now becomes the object for refraction at the retinoscopist's eye. Again, the first case is for a

16

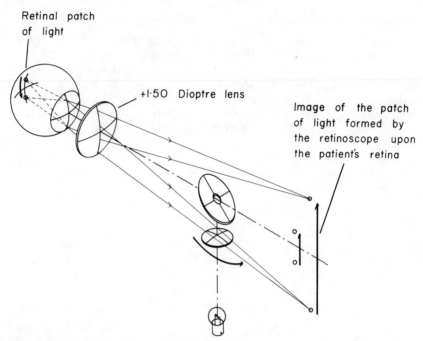

Retinal patch
of light

+1·50 Dioptre lens

Image of the patch
of light formed by
the retinoscope upon
the patient's retina

Figure 2.3. The formation of an aerial image of the retinal patch of light in a hyperope of less than 1.50 D. The arrows indicate the direction of movement of the image as the retinoscope's mirror is tilted down

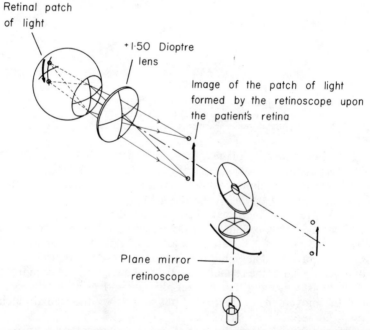

Retinal patch
of light

+1·50 Dioptre
lens

Image of the patch of light
formed by the retinoscope upon
the patient's retina

Plane mirror
retinoscope

Figure 2.4. The formation of an aerial image of the retinal patch of light in a myope. The arrows indicate the direction of movement of the image as the retinoscope's mirror is tilted down

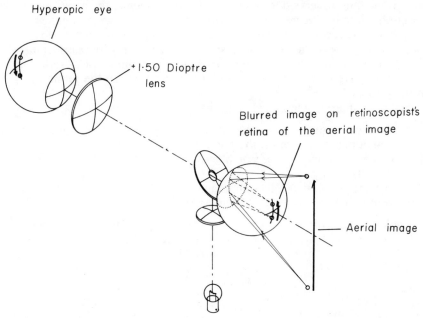

Figure 2.5. The formation, upon the retinoscopist's retina, of a blurred image of the aerial image in a hyoerope of less than 1.50 D. The arrows indicate the direction of movement of the image as the retinoscope's mirror is tilted down

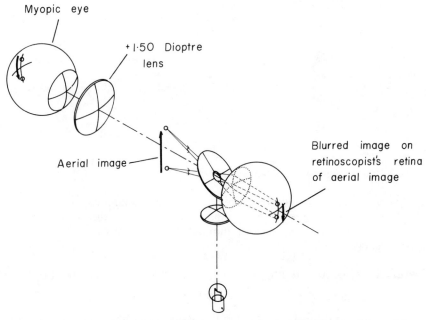

Figure 2.6. The formation, upon the retinoscopist's retina, of a blurred image of the aerial image in a myope. The arrows indicate the direction of movement of the image as the retinoscope's mirror is tilted down

hyperope and the second for a myope. It can be seen in the hyperopic case (*Figure 2.5*) that a blurred image of the aerial image is formed on the retina of the retinoscopist and that as the aerial image moves up so does the blurred image upon the retinoscopist's retina. In the myopic case a blurred image of the aerial image is again formed on the retinoscopist's retina, the difference here being that as the aerial image moves up the retinal image moves down.

So to summarize what has been said so far:

1. Downward movement of the mirror causes a downward movement of a small patch of light on the patient's retina;
2. An aerial image of this patch moves in the opposite direction, i.e. upwards;
3. The retinoscopist receives an image upon his or her retina that moves up in hyperopia and down in myopia.

Because the retinoscopist inverts everything seen on his or her retina, the reflex is seen as moving 'with' the movement of the mirror in hyperopia and 'against' the movement of the mirror in myopia.

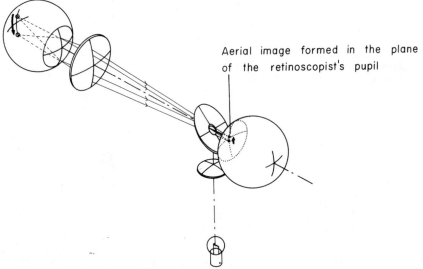

Aerial image formed in the plane of the retinoscopist's pupil

Figure 2.7. The point of reversal in retinoscopy

Figure 2.7 shows the point of reversal when the aerial image is formed in the plane of the retinoscopist's pupil. At this point, the whole of the retinoscopist's field of view is illuminated simultaneously, i.e. no movement is seen.

Determination of the axis of astigmatism with the retinoscope

Spot retinoscopy

The usual procedure with a spot retinoscope is to neutralize one of the principle meridians and then, by observing the more or less straight edge of the reflex patch seen in the pupil, to estimate the axis of the astigmatism.

Streak retinoscopy

There are two ways in which the axis of astigmatism can be measured with a streak retinoscope. The first is to focus the streak upon the patient's retina and then to rotate it until it is aligned with the bar of light that falls across the patient's face and pupil. This technique, which is not dissimilar to that of finding the axis of a spectacle lens by viewing a cross-line, can best be understood by considering what happens to the streak's image as it passes through the dioptrics of an astigmatic eye.

In *Figure 2.8* we have an immediate source of a streak retinoscope which is orientated at about 60 degrees to the horizontal meridian. The patient's

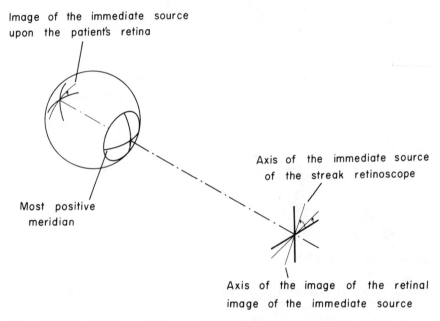

Image of the immediate source upon the patient's retina

Most positive meridian

Axis of the immediate source of the streak retinoscope

Axis of the image of the retinal image of the immediate source

Figure 2.8. The axis of the streak's image as it passes through the dioptrics of an astigmatic eye

eye is astigmatic, with the greatest positive power along the horizontal meridian. Because of the astigmatic nature of the patient's eye, the retinal image of the streak will be rotated towards the horizontal meridian. The optometrist views this image through the dioptrics of the patient's eye. In passing back through the astigmatic eye, the streak image will be rotated a second time towards the horizontal meridian. While looking at the patient's eye, the optometrist will see, therefore, a bar of light across the patient's iris and face at the same angle to the horizontal meridian as the immediate source, and a focused image of the streak, within the patient's pupil, at an angle much closer to the horizontal meridian (see *Figure 2.9(a)*). When the immediate source is aligned with one of the principal meridians of the astigmatic eye, then the central image (that within the pupil) will be aligned with the bar of light across the face (*see Figure 2.9(b)*).

The second technique of axis determination was described by Francis (1973). It is based upon the knowledge that rotation of a focused streak away from one of the principle meridians of the eye results in a thickening of its image. By looking for the position where the width of the streak is at a minimum, the axis of astigmatism can be found. Francis (1973) points out that the increase in thickness, as the line is rotated, is not the same for all

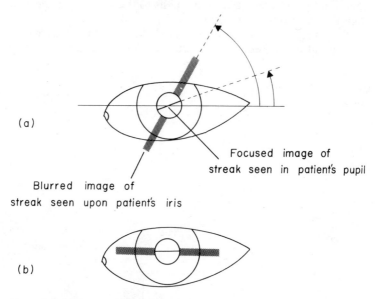

(a)

Focused image of
streak seen in patient's pupil

Blurred image of
streak seen upon patient's iris

(b)

Figure 2.9. (a) Appearance of the patient's eye when the streak is not lying along one of the principle meridians of the astigmatic eye. (b) Appearance of the patient's eye when the streak is lying along one of the principle meridians

refractive errors. The maximum increase in thickness, and therefore the greatest sensitivity, occurs when the eye is made artificially myopic by 1 D in its most hyperopic meridian and when the streak is focused along this meridian. This situation is easily obtained by:

1. Neutralizing the most hyperopic meridian;
2. Placing an additional +0.50 D lens in front of the patient's eye (this assumes that the retinoscopist is working at 66 cm);
3. Adjusting the vergence of light from the retinoscope until the line is focused along the meridian just neutralized.*

Instrument design

There are two broad categories of retinoscopes, spot retinoscopes and streak retinoscopes. The source of a spot retinoscope is an evenly

---

* With the Purvis streak retinoscope (Hamblin) the correct vergence is obtained with the focus adjusting lens in its lowest position.

illuminated circular patch of light, while that of a streak retinoscope is a single line that can be rotated around the axis of the instrument. This streak is usually produced by imaging a line filament bulb. Streak retinoscopes also allow the optometrist, via a knob which adjusts the position of the lens, to focus the source upon the retina of the patient. This control and the ability to rotate the source are used to determine the axis of astigmatism (*see* the previous section).

The mirrors used in retinoscopes are either semi-reflecting or have a small sight hole that enables the optometrist to view the reflex. The semi-reflecting mirrors lose a good proportion of the incident light, but have the advantage of not producing a shadow of the sight hole at the patient's eye.

Practitioners and students often find it difficult to decide which retinoscope to buy. There are no obvious optical differences between many of the instruments and there are no published reviews that offer assistance.† The choice is often, therefore, made on the instrument's mechanical construction (e.g. its styling, mechanical strength and whether or not it can be used by practitioners who wear spectacles), its expense and its availability. While it is true to say that today's standard of retinoscopes is of such a high order that reliable results can be obtained with virtually any instrument, there are certain important instrument parameters that affect the accuracy of retinoscopy. The next section briefly discusses some of these parameters.

The importance of certain instrument parameters upon the accuracy of retinoscopy

Hodd (1951) has described how particular instrument characteristics influence the accuracy of retinoscopy. He states that for the movement of the reflex to be easily identified, the edges of the reflex should be as sharp as possible and the movement slow. This can best be achieved by:

1. Keeping the sight hole small. As neutralization is approached, the reflex will be focused at or close to the observer's eye. Its image upon the retinoscopist's retina will be, therefore, out of focus. By reducing the size of the sight hole, we reduce the blurring of this image and hence sharpen its edges. Unfortunately, reducing the sight hole also decreases the brightness of the reflex. Some instruments, such as the Heine and American Optical streak retinoscopes, have a series of apertures that can be quickly changed by the optometrist. This allows the optometrist to opt for either a brighter reflex or a sharper edge to the reflex. In cases of patients with a hazy media, he or she may choose the larger sight hole in order to obtain a brighter reflex, while in normal patients where the reflex is fairly bright, the greater sensitivity that occurs with a smaller sight hole may be chosen.
2. Placing the immediate source fairly close to the mirror. This has two important effects. First, it will reduce the speed of the movement. The

† Sasieni (1979) has produced a survey of many of the currently manufactured instruments.

amount of movement of the immediate source, for any given rotation of the mirror, is proportional to its distance from the mirror. Second, the image of the source upon the patient's eye will, as neutralization is approached, be sharper. This in turn will produce a sharper reflex.

Hodd (1951) also points out that by keeping the size of the fundus patch small, the opposite edges of the reflex will be seen in quick succession, which aids recognition of reflex movement. This can best be achieved by keeping the source diameter small. Streak retinoscopes with line filament bulbs have, in effect, much smaller sources than equivalent spot retinoscopes and are better, therefore, at satisfying this criterion.

Errors in retinoscopy

A careful study into the differences between retinoscopy findings and subjective findings has been made by Millodot and O'Leary (1978). They found that the difference varied with age in the manner shown in *Figure 2.10*. In young people, retinoscopy gives a more positive estimation of the refractive error than subjective techniques. In old people the situation is reversed; retinoscopy gives a slightly more negative estimation of the refractive error.

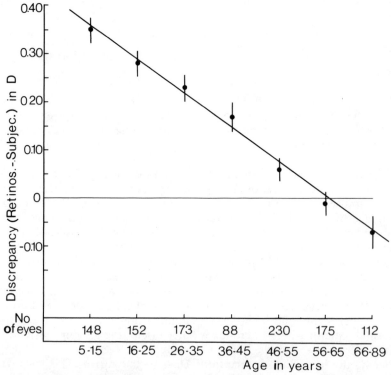

Figure 2.10. The average difference between retinoscopic and subjective (retinos. –subjec.) finding changes with age. From Millodot and O'Leary (1978), by permission of the authors and publishers

In an attempt to explain these findings, Millodot and O'Leary (1978) discussed four factors that could lead to a discrepancy between the two estimations of a refractive error:

1. The effect of alignment. It is impossible to be exactly along the line of sight of the patient in static retinoscopy. Thus, the refractive error is not measured at the fovea, but slightly to one side. According to Hodd (1948) the error due to misalignment is small as long as the retinoscopist does not go further than 8 degrees away from the line of sight;
2. Spherical aberration. The spherical aberration of the eye is in fact slight, predonimantly due to the flattening off of the radius of curvature of the cornea towards its periphery. It is not, therefore, a significant cause of error. Spherical aberration can, however, produce the situation where the movement of the reflex in the centre of the patient's pupil is seen to be different to that at the edges;
3. Chromatic aberration. Since the colour of the retinal reflex is red, retinoscopy will give a more hyperopic result than a subjective examination conducted with white light. Millodot and O'Leary (1980) claim that chromatic aberration can only account for part of the discrepancy between retinoscopic and subjective findings and that it cannot account for the variation in the discrepancy with age;
4. Site of reflex. An assumption is made in retinoscopy that the origin of the reflex coincides with the visual cells. If, in fact, the reflex were to originate from a surface in front of the visual cells, then a more positive finding would be made with the retinoscope. If, on the other hand, the reflex originated from a layer behind the visual cells, than a myopic error would be made.

Millodot and O'Leary (1978) explain their findings by suggesting that there are two layers within the retina that are responsible for the majority of the reflex, the internal limiting membrane and Bruch's membrane. These authors claim that in young people the reflex from the internal limiting membrane predominates and, because this layer is in front of the visual cells, a hyperopic error is made. As a person gets older so the reflective properties of this layer reduce along with its contribution to the reflex. In old age, the reflex comes predominantly from Bruch's membrane and so produces a slightly negative error. Evidence in support of their theory comes from examination of the fundi of young and old people. The fundi of young people are often seen to glisten, as though a layer in front of the retinal vessels reflects the ophthalmoscope light. Similar glistening is seen only rarely in older people.

Still further support for this theory comes from some earlier work done by Glickstein and Millodot (1970) on animals with differently sized eyes. They found that the smaller the eye, the greater was the degree of hyperopia measured with the retinoscope. Other techniques of refraction have shown these animals to be essentially emmetropic. If the reflex originates from in front of the visual cells then this finding can be explained because the dioptral equivalent of the same degree of movement within the retina will be greater for small eyes.

24   Retinoscopes

References

BENNETT, A. G. and FRANCIS, J. (1964). Retinoscopy and ophthalmoscopy. In *The Eye*, Vol. 4, ch. 10, p. 181. Edited by H. Davson. Academic Press, New York

BORISH, I. (1970). *Clinical Refraction*. The Professional Press, Chicago

DUKE-ELDER, S. (1970). *System of Ophthalmology*, Vol. 5. Henry Kimpton, London

EMSLEY, H. H. (1963). *Visual Optics*, Vol. 1, 5th Edn. Hatton Press, London

FRANCIS, J. (1973). The axis of astigmatism with special reference to streak retinoscopy. *British Journal of Physiological Optics*, **28,** 11

GLICKSTEIN, M. and MILLODOT, M. (1970). Retinoscopy and eye size. *Science*, **168,** 605

HODD, F. A. B. (1948). Retinoscopy. In *Some Recent Advances in Ophthalmic Optics. Transactions of the London Refraction Hospital Jubilee Congress 1947,* p. 146. Hatton Press, London

HODD, F. A. B. (1951). The measurement of spherical refraction by retinoscopy. In *Transactions of the International Optical Congress 1951*, p. 191. British Optical Association, London

MILLODOT, M. and O'LEARY, D. (1978). The discrepancy between retinoscopic and subjective measurements: Effects of age. *American Journal of Optometry and Physiological Optics,* **55,** 309

MILLODOT, M. and O'LEARY, D. (1980). On the artifact of retinoscopy and chromatic aberration. *American Journal of Optometry and Physiological Optics*, **57,** 822

SASIENI, L. S. (1979). A guide to retinoscopes. *Optician*, **177,** June 22nd, 17

3
Tonometers

Tonometers are instruments designed to evaluate the intraocular pressure. They are used by optometrists and ophthalmologists to assist in the diagnosis of glaucoma which, by definition, is a disease characterized by an increase in intraocular pressure. While intraocular pressure can be experimentally measured directly by cannulation (passing a small tube into the eye), it is estimated clinically by measuring either the degree of corneal deformation produced by a known weight or by measuring the weight needed to produce a given degree of deformation. Less deformation by a known weight, or a large weight required to produce a given deformation, is indicative of a high intraocular pressure. Attempts have been made to measure the intraocular pressure through the sclera, but the results tend to be erractic due to its non-uniformity and the added thickness of the conjunctiva and ciliary body.

Tonometers can be divided into those instruments that applanate, that is flatten, the cornea and those that indent it.

Applanation tonometers

Applanation tonometry is based upon the Imbert–Fick law which, when applied to the eye, states that the intraocular presssure (IOP) is equal to the tonometer weight divided by the applanated area (equation (3.1)).

$$IOP = \frac{\text{tonometer weight (g)}}{\text{applanated area (mm}^2)} \tag{3.1}$$

Strictly, this law is correct only for a spherical container, the limiting membrane of which is infinitely thin, perfectly flexible, elastic and dry. This type of membrane would create no resistance to flattening and, as the applanated area is increased, would allow expansion elsewhere so that the pressure within the container would not itself increase. The cornea satisfies none of these criteria. It is thick (0.5 mm) and has some structural rigidity which must be overcome by any applanating surface. It is also wet which allows a meniscus of tear fluid to form between the tonometer head and the eye. This meniscus creates a force that pulls the tonometer head towards the eye. Finally, the wall of the eye is not perfectly flexible and elastic, but has a rigidity. Thus, when a section of the eye is flattened the displaced fluid causes an elevation in the intraocular pressure. Even though the eye violates all these criteria, applanation tonometers can be made, with careful design, to closely approximate the Imbert–Fick law over the normal range of intraocular pressures and thus provide the clinician with a sufficiently accurate and useful tool.

Indentation tonometry

Indentation tonometry is based upon a simple relationship that states that the degree of indentation is proportional to the intraocular pressure (equation (3.2)).

$$\text{IOP} \propto \text{indentation (mm)} \tag{3.2}$$

As with applanation tonometry, the degree of indentation is dependent upon the flexibility of the cornea, surface tension forces and the elasticity of the walls of the eye. Again, careful design and calibration are required to ensure that the measurements do not give an inaccurate estimation of the intraocular pressure.

In order to translate either an applanation or indentation measurement into a value of intraocular pressure, calibration scales or tables are used (either incorporated in or provided with an instrument).

The calibration data are often obtained by using real or simulated eyes in which the pressure can be *directly* measured and varied (manometric studies). During this calibration procedure, certain normal values for variables such as ocular rigidity will have been assumed. Every tonometer is more or less sensitive to these variables and, therefore, may or may not produce significant measurement errors in individual measures. The better tonometers are those that are least affected by these variables and therefore record a measurement closer to the true intraocular pressure. Some instruments are calibrated against other tonometers, such as the Goldmann, in which accurate manometric calibration has already been achieved.

Normal range of IOP and factors that affect it

The average intraocular pressure is classically given as 15.5 mmHg with a normal range of 10–22 mmHg (Moses, 1975). The intraocular pressure is not constant within an individual, but varies according to the arterial pulse, whether the patient is erect or supine, and the time of day. The arterial pulse creates an oscillation in the intraocular pressure of about 2–3 mmHg (Quigley and Langham, 1975) and in going from an erect to a supine position the intraocular pressure increases by about 2–4 mmHg (Jain and Marmion, 1976a). The diurnal variation in intraocular pressure is normally about 5 mmHg, with maximum and minimum values occurring at any time during the day (Duke-Elder, 1952). However, the majority of people show a rise in the morning and a fall thereafter (Kitazawa and Horie, 1975; Horie and Kitazawa, 1979).

The diurnal range is dramatically increased in open-angle glaucoma; Horie and Kitazawa (1979) give an average value of 13.3 mmHg in a group of 39 open-angle glaucomatous patients, compared with 6.4 mmHg in a group of 21 normal patients. Duke-Elder (1952) investigated the phasic variations in the diurnal range in open-angle glaucoma and found that 55 per cent of patients have a rapidly rising pressure during morning, which peaks just before noon, falls to a trough in the early afternoon and is followed by a second rise at about 18.00 hours. A gradual rise in pressure throughout the day was shown by 25 per cent of patients, with peaks at about 16.00–18.00 hours, while the remaining 20 per cent gave the highest readings in the mornings, followed by a gradual decline throughout the day. Because of these varied patterns and the large range of intraocular pressures, many patients in the first stages of glaucoma have intraocular pressures within the normal range during some part of the day. As it is impossible to predict the exact time of day when the pressure is at its lowest, any single measurement that falls within the normal range cannot be interpreted with absolute certainty as indicating that the patient is not glaucomatous.

Types of statistics used in the clinical evaluations of tonometers

To evaluate tonometers researchers have used a variety of statistical techniques. To assist the reader to evaluate these studies, I have included in this section a brief account of the different types of statistics used and their relative merits.

Average differences

A statistic often given when two tonometers are compared is the average difference between their readings. For instance, an evaluator may say that, on average, tonometer X gives a reading 1 mmHg higher than tonometer Y. This statistic is useful to the clinician who is going to use the new tonometer because it will indicate at which readings the clinician should get suspicious of glaucoma. It does not, however, give any idea about the reliability of the readings taken with a given tonometer. For example, tonometer X may at one moment give readings very much higher than tonometer Y and the next moment give readings very much lower. If we assume that tonometer Y is accurate, then we must conclude that tonometer X is very inaccurate and unreliable, even though its *average* reading may be very close to that of tonometer Y. On the other hand, tonometer X may, on every measurement, give a reading 2 mmHg higher than tonometer Y, in which case the tonometer is very reliable, but has a significant average difference.

Average values are therefore useful when other statistical data are given about a particular tonometer. In isolation, average values are of little value.

Correlation coefficient

This statistic gives an estimate of the degree of closeness of a linear relationship between two tonometers. It we take our two tonometers X and Y, then the correlation coefficient will tell us how well the results from the tonometer under evaluation, X, compare with the results from our standard tonometer, Y. If there is a perfect correlation between X and Y – that is, if we always obtain the same reading with tonometer X that we do with tonometer Y – then the correlation coefficient will be 1. If there is absolutely no relationship between the readings taken with tonometers X and Y, then the coefficient will be approximately 0.

The correlation coefficient is designed to be independent of the units of measure. It can be used to give an estimate of the dependence of a person's weight on his height just as well as an estimate of the closeness of a relationship between the measurements given by two tonometers. Because of this we find that if, as in our previous example, a tonometer *always* gives a reading 2 mmHg higher than the standard its correlation coefficient will still be 1, as there is a perfect correlation between the two instruments even though they never give the same reading. The same situation applies if tonometer X always gives a reading that is, say, one-half that of tonometer Y.

Another point to realize about this statistic is that it can vary with the range of pressures used in the sample. If an evaluator chooses a normal group of subjects whose intraocular pressures range from 15 mmHg to 20 mmHg, then a higher correlation coefficient may be obtained than if a group was chosen that incorporated some glaucomatous subjects and had a range from 15 mmHg to 40 mmHg.

This does not mean that the evaluator who chooses a normal group unfairly biases the results in the favour of the instrument being evaluated. In optometry, a tonometer only needs to be accurate in the range of suspicious intraocular pressures. Once outside this range, its accuracy is of less importance. For example, if a tonometer reads 45 mmHg instead of 40 or 35 mmHg instead of 40, the patient would still be referred with suspect glaucoma. This sort of error cannot be tolerated, however, in the suspicious range of intraocular pressures (20–25 mmHg) because it could result in a serious misdiagnosis. Ideally, correlation coefficients should be given for intraocular pressures that straddle the suspicious range. In ophthalmology, a greater range of accuracy may be desirable in order to assess the effectiveness of different forms of treatment in reducing the intraocular pressure.

One final point to be made is that the variability of intraocular pressure measurements with time means that even when the same tonometer is used to give both X and Y values, the correlation coefficient will not equal 1. Moses and Liu (1968) have shown that repeated measurements with the Goldmann tonometer differ by more than 2 mmHg in 35 per cent of readings. If the correlation coefficient had been calculated, it would have been less than 1.

The standard deviation of the differences

The standard deviation of the differences gives an estimation of the variance between the readings taken with two tonometers. If the standard deviation of the differences is given as 2 mmHg, this means that 68 per cent of the results obtained with two tonometers differ by 2 mmHg or less. The lower the value, the less is the variance between the two instruments. If one of the set of readings is taken as being the true intraocular pressure, then the standard deviation of the differences tells us how accurate the second tonometer is.

The standard deviation of the differences operates in a similar way to the correlation coefficient in that if one tonometer always reads a constant amount higher or lower than another, then the standard deviation of the differences (SD) will give no variance between the results (SD = 0). It differs from the correlation coefficient in that if a linear relationship exists between the two tonometers, such as in the example given before where tonometer X always gives a reading equal to one-half that of tonometer Y, the linear relationship will not be recognized by this SD statistic, which may give a very high value for the standard deviation of the differences.

The standard deviation of the differences may be, to some extent, dependent upon the range of intraocular pressures used in the evaluation. For optometric purposes, the ideal range should be made to straddle the suspicious range of intraocular pressures.

Ideally, researchers who evaluate tonometers should give at least two different statistical measures – the first should give an estimate of the variance between the two measurements and the second should give the relationship between the two measurements. Unfortunately, not all researchers have done this. While an attempt is made in the following discussions of tonometers to select evaluations in which careful statistical analysis has been done, this has not always been possible because of lack of published data. The reader should, therefore, be careful in going through this review not to judge a particular tonometer on the basis of an isolated statistical measure.

The Schiotz tonometer

The Schiotz indentation tonometer was first designed in 1905 and has undergone little change since its invention. The instrument measures the degree of corneal indentation produced by a known weight that rests upon the cornea. The plunger assembly (*see Figure 3.1*) provides the indenting force to the cornea and can be set at either 5.5 g, 7.5 g, 10 g or 15 g by the addition of small weights. The concave footplate assembly, which rests upon the cornea, forms a reference level from which the plunger further indents the cornea. The total weight supported by the cornea is 16.5 g (with the 5.5 g plunger assembly). The degree of indentation produced by the plunger assembly is displayed on the scale of the instrument; each division of the scale represents 1/20 mm of indentation. This scale measurement can be converted into mmHg by the use of tables, of which the most commonly used is that developed by Friedenwald (1957). His table is based upon manometric readings and assumes that the eye being measured has an average ocular rigidity.

If a patient has a normal pressure and a very rigid eye, then the indentation produced by the plunger assembly will be less than that seen in a patient with the same intraocular pressure and an eye of normal rigidity. The extrapolated intraocular pressure of the first patient will be recorded as being higher than the true intraocular pressure. Conversely, if a patient has a high intraocular pressure and an eye of low rigidity, then the extrapolated intraocular pressure will be recorded as being less than the true intraocular pressure. The magnitude of these errors can be substantial

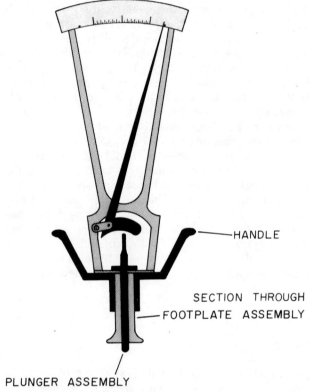

HANDLE

SECTION THROUGH
FOOTPLATE ASSEMBLY

PLUNGER ASSEMBLY

Figure 3.1. The Schiotz tonometer

due to the relatively large amount of fluid displaced by the tonometer when it is placed upon the eye. To try and overcome this problem, Friedenwald devised a nomogram (*see Figure 3.2*) for the Schiotz tonometer which allows the clinician to compensate for the effect of an abnormal ocular rigidity. To utilize the nomogram it is necessary to have a scale reading with at least two different plunger weights. Unfortunately, there are difficulties in reading the tonometer scale with sufficient accuracy to make the nomogram reliable. Errors of only one-half a scale division, which have relatively little effect upon the intraocular presssure reading obtained from the tables, can have a very significant effect upon the extrapolated pressure from the nomogram (Gloster, 1965). This problem cannot be overcome by taking a series of readings with the Schiotz tonometer because with each measurement the intraocular pressure is reduced due to the weight of the tonometer, which increases the outflow of aqueous from the eye.

The rather excessive weight of the Schiotz indentation tonometer (16.5 g) is prone to cause more corneal damage than many of the applanation tonometers, which only exert a force of a few grams against the cornea. The cornea is particularly prone to damage if the tonometer is slid around during the measurement process. The likelihood of this is

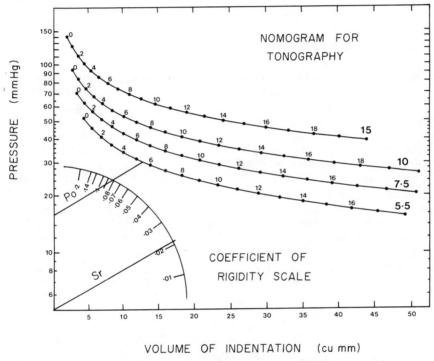

Figure 3.2. Fridenwald's nomogram for the Schiotz tonometer. The line Po is drawn through the two scale readings taken with different weights of the tonometer. The line Sr, which gives a measurement of the coefficient of rigidity, is drawn parallel to the line Po and through the origin

increased by the fact that the scale reading has to be made while the tonometer is in contact with the eye. Despite these problems, the Schiotz indentation tonometer is still one of the most widely used instruments for the estimation of intraocular pressure. Its low cost, simplicity of design, mechanical reliability and availability has made it attractive to many optometric practices.

Various forms of electronically recording Schiotz tonometers are now available. These instruments are used in tonography, which is a technique for measuring the facility of outflow of aqueous humour from the eye. When the Schiotz tonometer is placed upon the cornea, it artificially raises the intraocular pressure. In the normal eye, this increased pressure results in an increased rate of outflow of the aqueous through the angle of the anterior chamber and a consequent reduction in the measured intraocular pressure. The rate of fall of the intraocular pressure is related to the facility of the outflow of aqueous from the eye. In tonography, the pressure is continuously recorded over a period of 4 min. The outflow over this time is measured in mm^3 (cu mm) by using a series of equations developed by Friedenwald. Values of less than 0.11 mm^3 are almost always indicative of glaucoma. Unfortunately, tonography is most reliable in severe, well established cases of glaucoma. In borderline cases, the variability in results is high and thus the reliability low (Gloster, 1965).

The Goldmann tonometer

The Goldmann tonometer measures the force required to applanate the cornea over a circular area of diameter 3.06 mm, a value chosen for three reasons. First, the amount of fluid displaced with such a small applanated area is negligible (approximately 0.5 $\mu\ell$). This means that the intraocular pressure during measurement is practically identical to the true intraocular pressure, even though the walls of the eye have some rigidity. Second, Goldmann has shown, from studies on enucleated eyes, that for an applanation area of diameter 3–4 mm the surface tension force that results from the corneal film is equal, but opposite, to the force required to counteract corneal rigidity. Thus, the tonometer force becomes equal to the intraocular pressure. Finally, when a diameter of 3.06 mm is used, the (tonometer force in g × 10) is equal to the force in mmHg, i.e. a simple conversion.

In order to measure the intraocular pressure the entire tonometer, which is composed of an applanating head and a spring-loaded lever, is attached

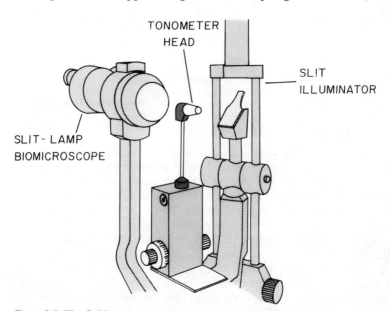

Figure 3.3. The Goldmann tonometer attached to a Haag–Streit slit lamp

to a slit lamp (*see Figure 3.3*). The head is brought into contact with the anaesthetized cornea by gradually moving the slit-lamp body towards the patient. When contact is made, the optometrist views the applanated area, which is made visible by the instillation of some fluorescein, through the microscope and applanating head. The pressure exerted against the eye is then adjusted with the spring-loaded lever until the applanated area has a diameter of 3.06 mm.

To facilitate accurate recording, two prisms with their bases in opposite directions are placed within the head. These prisms split the applanated area into two and separate the two half images by 3.06 mm (*see Figure 3.4*). The optometrist sees two semi-circles, as shown in *Figure 3.5*. When the two inside edges are just touching, the applanated area has the correct diameter. Care must be taken during measurement to establish that the applanated area is bisected by the dividing line between the two prisms. Failure to do this can result in a slight error in the recorded intraocular pressure.

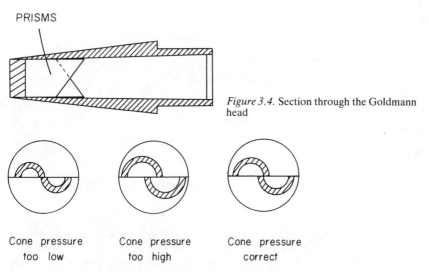

PRISMS

Figure 3.4. Section through the Goldmann head

Cone pressure   Cone pressure   Cone pressure
too low   too high   correct

Figure 3.5. View through the Goldmann tonometer head. The shaded areas are the tear menisci made visible by the installation of fluorescein and illumination with ultraviolet light

American Optical have recently developed a new type of tonometer head that does away with the need for this accurate vertical alignment. Their system utilizes a biprism to double the image of the applanated area, rather than the two prisms contained within the Haag–Steit (H–S) head. The doubling biprism is not contained within the head, but placed just in front of the microscope's objective, as shown in *Figure 3.6*. Koester, Campbell and Dunn (1980), who describe the system in full, point out that, with experienced ophthalmologists, there is no difference in the results obtained with the two types of doubling systems, although when first using this type of tonometer it may be easier to use the American Optical head.

Moses and Liu (1968) assessed the consistency of the Goldmann tonometer by taking two sets of measurements on 148 eyes. They found that repeated measurements differed by 2 mmHg or more in 35 per cent of cases. They ascribed this difference to real changes of the intraocular pressure.

When repeated measurements of the intraocular pressure are taken with the Goldmann tonometer, the intraocular pressure is found to gradually fall by about 3–4 mmHg over a period of 5 min. In the contralateral eye there is a sympathetic fall in intraocular pressure. The exact mechanism of this phenomenon is still obscure, but it has been shown by Krakau and

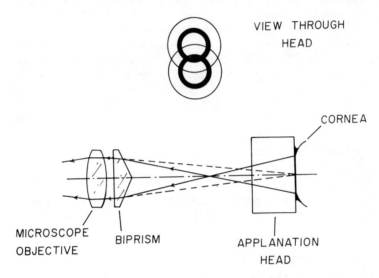

Figure 3.6. A new type of tonometer head for the Goldmann tonometer (American Optical)

Wilke (1971) to be partially dependent upon the weight of the tonometer against the eye. When a vibration tonometer was used, the loaded weight of which was only 0.1 g, they found a fall in intraocular pressure of only 0.4 mmHg over a period of 5 min, compared with a 2.9 mmHg fall when the Goldmann was used. Increasing the weight of the vibration tonometer to 0.3 g and 0.6 g resulted in falls of 1.1 mmHg and 1.5 mmHg, respectively.

The Goldmann tonometer has, over the years, become the standard to which all other tonometers are compared. Its accuracy in manometric studies is excellent (Moses, 1958). Its simplicity of design, rugged nature and ease of sterilization has made it the obvious choice for many optometric practices. While Goldmann tonometry is taken as the standard to which all other tonometers are compared, errors due to misuse can and often do arise with this instrument. Some of the common ones are:

1. Lids touch the probe – results in a high reading;
2. Surface tension of tears altered by the use of liquids other than water to wet the fluorets – this effect is minimal;

3. Improper cleaning of the head – it must have standard wetting characteristics;
4. Corneal astigmatism – in instances of high astigmatism, the flattest meridian should be placed at 43 degrees to the axis of the cone;
5. Meniscus width too wide – should be as narrow as possible.

A hand-held version of the Goldmann tonometer has been developed by Perkins (1965) (*see Figure 3.7*). This instrument, which utilizes a spring to exert a variable pressure upon the eye, can be used equally well whether the patient is supine or erect. Dunn and Brubaker (1973) examined two

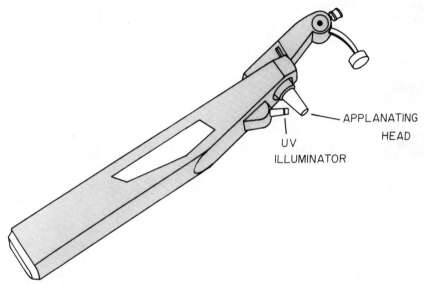

Figure 3.7. The Perkins hand-held tonometer (Clement Clark)

commercially produced versions of this tonometer in the laboratory. They found that the spring arrangement gave excellent linearity over the operating range of the instrument when the instrument was used either horizontally, such as on a supine patient, or vertically. Their only criticism was that the zero position of one of the instruments tested was 0.75 mmHg out, such that it always measured 0.75 mmHg above the true intraocular pressure.

Clinical evaluations of the Perkins tonometer have been conducted by Wallace and Lovell (1968) and Whitty (1969), who report excellent correlation with the slit-lamp mounted Goldmann. They also reported that patients prefer the hand-held tonometer and that, with a little practice, it is as easy to use as the slit-lamp mounted version. Its other obvious advantage is that of being portable.

The Applanometer and Tonomat applanation tonometers

The Tonomat was developed in the US in 1967. It differs from its predecessor, the Applanometer, by having disposable endplates and a slightly different shaped handle. While of these two only the Tonomat is readily available today, the clinical evaluations of the Applanometer bear relevance to the Tonomat and are included in the following discussion.

The Tonomat instrument, shown in *Figure 3.8*, uses the principle of applying a constant tonometer weight to the cornea and then measuring the applanated area. The larger the applanated area, the lower the intraocular pressure. When in use, the disposable endplates are first covered with a thin film of Argyrol stain, which is a brown, sticky

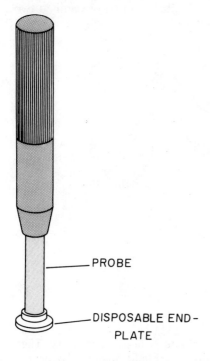

PROBE

DISPOSABLE END-
PLATE

Figure 3.8. The Tonomat tonometer

substance usually applied to the endplate with the aid of a cotton-wool bud. The patient, whose cornea has been anaesthetized, is put in a supine position face towards the ceiling. The tonometer endplate is lowered onto the cornea until the total weight (5 g) of the stainless steel probe and endplate is supported by the cornea, the probe weight being free to slide up and down within the handle. The instrument is then lifted vertically away from the cornea. An estimation of the intraocular pressure is obtained by measuring the area over which the stain has been removed from the endplate by the applanated cornea. The instrument comes with an eyepiece measuring device that enables the applanated area to be directly converted into mmHg.

The calibration scale used with the Applanometer and Tonomat instruments was developed by Posner and Inglima (1962a, b), largely on the basis of paired readings between the Applanometer and Goldmann tonometers. The Applanometer has been clinically evaluated by Gloster and Martin (1965) who compared it with the Goldmann and an electronic Schiotz tonometer (Schwarzer). They reported that the Applanometer tended to overestimate pressures below 26 mmHg and underestimate pressures over 26 mmHg. The correlation coefficient for the Applanometer and Goldmann was 0.80, while that for the Goldmann and Schiotz was 0.88. Their conclusions were that the Applanometer was no more accurate than the Schiotz tonometer, although it was influenced less by scleral rigidity.

There are at least three sources of potential error when using the Applanometer or Tonomat instruments. First, if the weight is lowered a little too fast, then a large, transient area of applanation exists which results in the measured pressure being below the true intraocular pressure. Second, the area of the endplate over which the dye is removed includes the tear meniscus, which results in the estimated intraocular pressure being partly dependent upon the amount of tears within the eye. Finally, if the tonometer is moved or if the eye moves while the endplate is in contact with the cornea, the dye will be removed over an area larger than that applanated. If the movement is only in one meridian, the area on the endplate that is devoid of dye will be elliptical and a valid measurement can still be made by measuring along the shortest dimension. If, however, the movement is in more than one meridian then the recorded intraocular pressure will be less than the true intraocular pressure.

Although these instruments are possibly no more accurate than the Schiotz, they are much easier to sterilize and less liable to abrade the cornea. In addition to this, they are relatively cheap and are mechanically very reliable because of their simple design.

The Mackay–Marg tonometer

The Mackay–Marg tonometer is an electronic instrument that was developed in the early 1960s within the US. At that time, optometrists in the US were not allowed to use anaesthetics and one of the objectives of Mackay and Marg was to develop a tonometer that could be used on the unanaesthetized eye. Today, however, the instrument is rarely used without an anaesthetic.

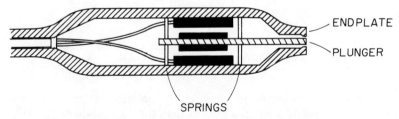

Figure 3.9. Section through the probe of the Mackay–Marg tonometer

The Mackay–Marg tonometer is composed of two main parts, a probe and a recording amplifier. The probe, which is shown in detail in *Figure 3.9*, is composed of a central, stainless steel plunger supported within a magnetic field by two springs. The tip of the plunger protrudes by a very small amount (5 microns) from the endplate. Movement of the plunger with respect to the endplate generates an electrical signal within the probe body that is transmitted to the amplifier and recorded on a strip chart.

The operating principles of the instrument are shown in *Figure 3.10.* When the probe is first brought into contact with the cornea the plunger is pushed back with respect to the endplate. This movement of the plunger produces a positive deflection of the needle on the strip chart. The degree of movement of the plunger is dependent upon the sum of at least two forces – the intraocular pressure and the force necessary to bend the

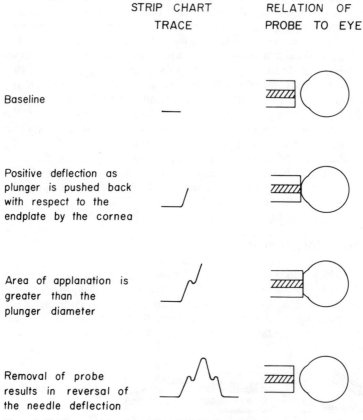

Figure 3.10. The operating principles of the Mackay–Marg tonometer

cornea. As the probe is advanced, the area of applanation increases until the cornea is flattened over an area greater than the plunger diameter. It is claimed that a point is eventually reached when the force necessary to bend the cornea is supported wholly by the endplate. The removal of this force from the plunger allows it to move forward slightly and a small, negative deflection is seen on the strip chart. Advancing the probe still further increases the intraocular pressure and pushes the probe further back into the endplate, which results in a second positive deflection of the strip chart needle.

The bottom of the small trough produced when the corneal bending force is taken over by the endplate is believed to be related solely to the intraocular pressure. Measurement of the height of this trough from the baseline allows the intraocular pressure to be estimated. Removal of the probe from the eye results in a reversal of the needle deflection pattern seen during the period when the probe was advanced. The whole process involves contact with the eye for no more than a second or two, which is one reason why the measurement can be taken on the unanaesthetized eye.

Manometric studies with the Mackay–Marg tonometer have been conducted by Moses, Marg and Oechsli (1962) and Hilton and Shaffer (1966). Both sets of results show a good correlation between manometric pressure and the height of the trough on the strip chart. Two independent clinical evaluations of the Mackay–Marg tonometer have been made, one by Tierney and Rubin (1966) and the other by Hilton and Shaffer (1966).

Tierney and Rubin compared the Mackay–Marg with the Goldmann and Schiotz tonometers. They found (using anaesthetics) that the Mackay–Marg gave results, on average, 2 mmHg higher than the Goldmann and Schiotz instruments. The correlation coefficient between the results of the Mackay–Marg and Goldmann tonometers was 0.93. This result was obtained from a sample of 248 eyes which contained both normal and glaucomatous patients. The instrument was found to have a higher standard deviation of results on normal eyes than the Goldmann and Schiotz tonometers; 3.5 vs 2.83 and 2.98, respectively. Tierney and Rubin (1966) point out that this will indicate a larger range of suspect intraocular pressures in the normal population and a subsequent tendency to refer a larger number of normal patients. They also reported that errors in application of the instrument tended to give higher measures of the intraocular pressure than the true one. False positives are therefore more likely than false negatives.

Hilton and Shaffer (1966) found that the Mackay–Marg gave a value, on average, 1 mmHg higher than the Goldmann and a correlation coefficient of 0.99 on 64 eyes, the majority of which were within the normal range of intraocular pressures. They reported that the practitioner should always take the lowest of a series of readings as probe misalignment or a spasm of the orbicularis produces artifically high readings. They conclude by saying that while the instrument has some advantages over the Goldmann, such as not requiring a slit lamp and allowing measurements with the patient in any position, its disadvantages (high cost, complexity) mean that it is of little asset to the ophthalmologist. The change of the laws that relate to the use of anaesthetics within the US and the now more common appearance of slit lamps in optometric practices means that Hilton and Shaffer's comments apply equally well to many optometric practices.

The Tonair tonometer

The Tonair tonometer is a hand-held instrument which measures the intraocular pressure in terms of air pressure. The instrument is composed to two main parts; a probe and an amplifier recorder.

The probe contains a small, moveable plunger that protrudes from the endplate when not in contact with the eye (*see Figure 3.11*). A small electronic pump, situated within the amplifier recorder, delivers a constant flow of air into the probe chamber via a flexible tube. This air is allowed to escape through small vents in the side of the probe as long as the plunger is in the forward position. When the probe is brought into contact with the cornea the plunger is pushed back into the endplate where it acts as a

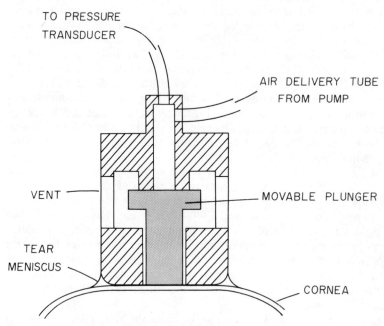

TO PRESSURE
TRANSDUCER

AIR DELIVERY TUBE
FROM PUMP

VENT

MOVABLE PLUNGER

TEAR
MENISCUS

CORNEA

Figure 3.11. Section through the probe of the Tonair tonometer

valve, thus cutting off communication between the air chamber and the vents. The chamber pressure thus gradually rises and exerts an increasing force against the plunger. As soon as the chamber pressure exceeds the counterpressure exerted by the deformed cornea, the plunger moves downwards and the air is allowed to escape. The extent of the downward movement is of the order of 0.025 mm. The pressure within the chamber required to move the plunger is related to the intraocular pressure and is recorded by a transducer situated within the amplifier recorder.

Since the corneal bending takes place at the periphery of the probe, the central plunger (diameter 2 mm) is not affected by the cornea's structural rigidity. Likewise, the surface tension forces created by the tear meniscus act solely upon the probe body. It is therefore claimed that the only force that acts upon the plunger is that of the intraocular pressure (Steinberg and Adise, 1964).

Manometric studies, using an inflated rubber balloon, have been conducted by Steinberg and Adise (1964). Their results show a good correlation between the tonometer readout and the manometer gauge. The value of this finding is limited, due to the marked differences between a rubber balloon and the human eye.

Clinical evaluations of the tonometer have been undertaken by both Steinberg (1965) and Posner and Inglima (1968). Steinberg (1965) compared the Tonair with the Goldmann, Schiotz and Applanometer tonometers in three separate studies. He found a good correlation between the Tonair and the other three instruments, although the Tonair's results were, on average, 1 mmHg higher than the Goldmann's and 2 mmHg higher than those of the Schiotz. The correlation coefficient between the Goldmann and the Tonair was 0.81 for 60 eyes, the majority of which fell within the normal range of intraocular pressures.

Posner and Inglima (1968), who undertook a study of the Tonair for the Committee of Standardization of Tonometers of the American Academy of Ophthalmology and Otolaryngology, did not obtain such good results. They compared the Tonair with the Schiotz and Applanometer tonometers. They found a much greater scatter of results in the Tonair *vs.* Schiotz and the Tonair *vs.* Applanometer scatter grams than in the Schiotz *vs.* Applanometer. They concluded that the increased scatter was the result of the Tonair tonometer.

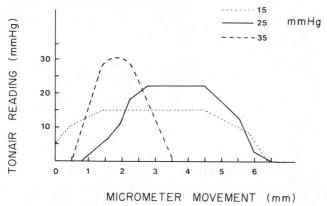

Figure 3.12. Effect of probe misalignment. The plateau of each curve represents the central region of the membrane where identical measurements were obtained. The sloping segment on each side shows the degree to which the pressure is underestimated when the probe is applied off centre. From Posner and Inglima (1968) by permission of the author and publishers

In addition to their clinical survey, Posner and Inglima (1968) also investigated the effect of probe misalignment upon the recorded intraocular pressure using an inflated rubber drum. They found that when the tonometer is normally applied to an eccentric part of the drum, the reading obtained may be considerably below the manometric pressure. They also found that the area of the drum over which consistent results are obtained decreases with increasing drum pressure (*see Figure 3.12*). It can be seen from this figure that at a pressure of 35 mmHg, a 1 mm displacement from the centre produces a drastic reduction in the measured pressure. It is generally believed that at a pressure of 35 mmHg, the accuracy required to obtain repeatable and accurate results is greater than can be reasonably expected from a hand-held instrument. When measuring high intraocular pressures, therefore, there is a serious likelihood of recording a value below the true intraocular pressure. This means that the instrument, rather than being a fail-safe device, like the Mackay–Marg instrument which records a higher-than-true intraocular pressure when the probe is mis-aligned with the cornea, is one that tends to record normal pressures in patients with elevated intraocular pressures.

The Pneuma-tonometer

The Pneuma-tonometer has undergone several name changes throughout its development. It was originally called the Durham–Langham tonometer and then the Applamatic.

The Pneuma-tonometer, like other electronic tonometers, is composed of two parts; a probe and an amplifier recorder. The probe (*see Figure 3.13*) is about 15 cm long and is connected to the amplifier recorder by two gas-tight, flexible tubes. One of these tubes delivers the gas at a constant

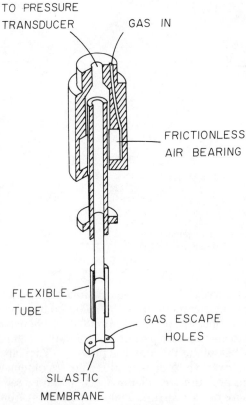

Figure 3.13. Section through the probe of the Pneuma-tonometer (Digilab)

rate into the chamber of the probe while the other tube connects the probe chamber to a pressure transducer situated within the amplifier recorder. The tip of the probe is connected to the chamber of the cone via a tube; thus the pressure within the tip is equal to that recorded by the transducer.

When used on the eye, the Silastic membrane of the probe is placed against the cornea where it adopts the convex shape of the cornea and occludes the small holes in the tip. The pressure within the chamber gradually increases until the cornea is applanated by the Silastic membrane and the air is allowed to escape through the holes. Once this point has been reached, the intraocular pressure is continuously recorded by the tonometer, the current value being displayed digitally or permanently recorded on a continuous strip chart. Continuous recording is made possible because the piston floats on a frictionless air bearing. Without this bearing, small hand tremors would result in an erratic measurement of the intraocular pressure. The early versions of this tonometer (the Durham–Langham) did not incorporate this bearing and consequently could not record continuously. The small flexible coupling near the tip allows it to align itself with the corneal surface. An example of the strip chart output is given in *Figure 3.14*. The ocular pulse can be seen clearly on this recording.

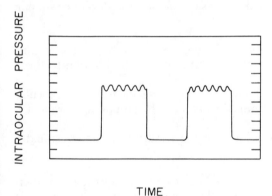

TIME

Figure 3.14. Strip chart output of the Pneuma-tonometer which shows two separate applications of the probe to the eye. The ripple in the recording during the time that the probe is on the eye is due to the ocular pulse

The Pneuma-tonometer exerts a force of some 2 g against the cornea. This can be increased, for tonography, by the application of small weights to the tip. The addition of these weights does not affect the instrument's ability to record continuously.

The instrument has been clinically evaluated by both Quigley and Langham (1975) and Jain and Marmion (1976b). Quigley and Langham (1975) measured the intraocular pressure with both the Goldmann and Pneuma-tonometer in normal and glaucomatous eyes. They found that the Pneuma-tonometer gave slightly higher readings than the Goldmann. When using the later and more accurate calibration, they found that the number of people in whom the difference in intraocular pressure reading between the two tonometers was greater than 2 mmHg was almost identical to that reported by Moses and Liu (1968) for repeat measurements with the Goldmann. They concluded that the differences between the two instruments could be explained by the normal fluctuations in intraocular pressure. No measurements of the correlation coefficient or standard deviation of the differences were given in this evaluation.

Jain and Marmion (1976b) also compared the results obtained with the Pneuma-tonometer with those from a Goldmann tonometer in both normal and glaucomatous populations. They found that, on average, the Pneuma-tonometer gave readings 0.75 mmHg higher than the Goldmann in normal patients and 1.25 mmHg higher in glaucomatous patients, the difference between the two tonometers tending to increase with the higher pressures. In general, they found that the instrument gave intraocular pressure readings of an accuracy comparable with that of the Goldmann. They also point out that it has the advantage over the Goldmann of being portable, being able to measure independently of the posture of the patient and being able to perform tonography. No measures of the variance between the Goldmann and Penuma-tonometer were given.

A less favourable laboratory evaluation has been given by Moses and Grodzki (1979). They performed a series of manometric studies on human eyes and found the following:

1. The Pneuma-tonometer probe is position sensitive – the results obtained with the probe vertical were found to be different to those with it horizontal;
2. It is not suitable for tonography because the measured intraocular pressure is grossly underestimated when the 10 g tonography weight is added to the probe;
3. It overestimates the lower intraocular pressures and underestimates the higher ones.

Moses and Grodzki (1979) do not give the correlation coefficients for their data, although from their scatter plots these would appear to be very close to 1. If this is correct it should, by altering the calibration scales of the tonometer, be possible to obtain accurate and reliable measurements of the intraocular pressure with this tonometer.

The American Optical non contact tonometer

The non contact tonometer (NCT) (*see Figure 3.15*), was designed and developed by Grolman (1972). It heralds a totally new concept in tonometry as it does not require any contact to be made between the tonometer and the eye. Intraocular pressure measurements can therefore be taken without an anaesthetic. The instrument operates by sending a puff of air toward the cornea with more than sufficient strength to momentarily applanate it. The point of applanation is detected by an optical system. The time taken from the onset of the puff to the applanation of the cornea is

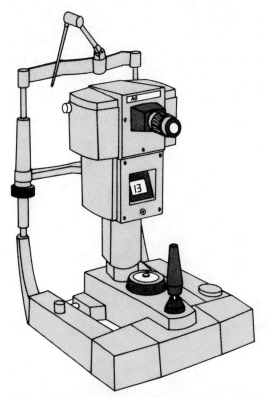

Figure 3.15. The American Optical non contact tonometer

recorded electronically and has been found to be related to the intraocular pressure.

   The puff of air is produced by a piston, within a cylinder, being rapidly moved by a solenoid. The compressed air within the chamber escapes, via a tube, onto the patient's cornea (*see Figure 3.16*). The pressure of the air that escapes from the tube increases linearly with time over a peri d of 10 ms, as shown in *Figure 3.17*. After this time the pressure falls off again.

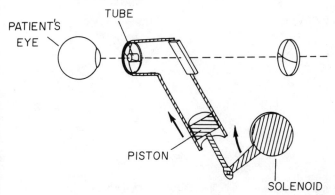

Figure 3.16. Section through the air chamber of the non contact tonometer

The pressure exerted by the puff on the cornea is sufficiently great to indent it over a small central region. In passing from its normal convex shape to one of concavity, this region of the cornea goes through a stage where it is approximately applanated. The point of applanation is detected by a collimated light source and a detector. The collimated light source projects a beam of light at the corneal vertex while the detector receives the reflected light from the cornea. When the corneal vertex is convex or concave, the amount of light that falls on the detector is very small.

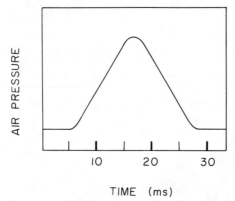

Figure 3.17. Graph of the air pressure that leaves the tube versus time

However, when it is flat, i.e. applanated, the detector signal increases (*see Figure 3.18*). The time taken from the onset of the puff to when the output of the detector reaches a maximum is recorded electronically. This time is a measure of the pressure needed to applanate the cornea and is directly related to the intraocular pressure. The electronic circuitry within the tonometer processes the time signal and digitally displays the computed intraocular pressure.

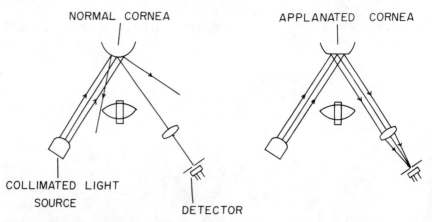

Figure 3.18. An increased amount of light falls upon the detector when the cornea is applanated

Because it is important that the puff be directed at the vertex of the cornea and that the instrument be placed at an exact distance from the cornea, an optical alignment system is incorporated within the instrument. This system is similar to that used within a radiuscope and it permits alignment along all three axes. In addition to the operator alignment system, there is an automatic alignment verification system. If alignment is not correct at the time of the puff then the result is not displayed, which makes a repeat measurement necessary. Details of the optical and automatic alignment systems are shown in *Figure 3.19.*

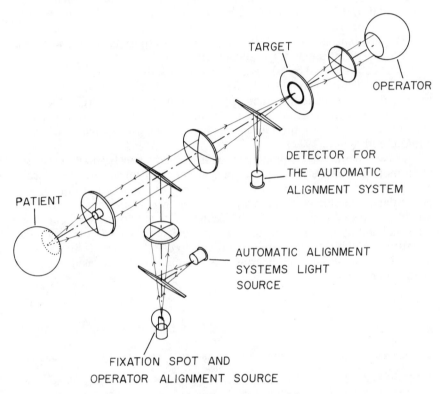

Figure 3.19. The operator and automatic alignment systems of the non contact tonometer

Single measurements of the intraocular pressure are not very reliable with the NCT. Variations of the order of 3–4 mmHg are common due to the cardiac cycle, but this problem can be overcome by taking repeated measures. When the mean of three measurement is used rather than a single measurement, the results become very consistent (Myers and Scott, 1975).

Calibration of this instrument has been achieved from clinical studies (Forbes, Pico and Grolman, 1974) on both glaucomatous and normal subjects in which the results of the NCT were compared with those of the Goldmann. For the purposes of calibration, the Goldmann was assumed to be error-free. The calibration results give the standard deviation of differences between the Goldmann and the NCT as 2.86 mmHg. Normal physiological changes in the intraocular pressure can account for much of this variability (Moses and Liu, 1968).

An independent clinical evaluation of the NCT has been conducted by Burman (1974) in which he compares the NCT with the Mackay–Marg tonometer. He found a very good correlation between the two instruments (correlation coefficient 0.87); the Mackay–Marg gave, on average, an intraocular pressure measurement 1 mmHg higher than that of the NCT. The higher average reading with the Mackay–Marg instrument may, in part, be due to the measurements being taken without an anaesthetic (Rosenthal and Werner, 1969). The accuracy of the NCT in measuring intraocular pressures above 35 mmHg has been questioned by Sorensen (1975). This inaccuracy is of little importance to optometrists as it is well above the normal range of intraocular pressures.

It has been reported by Myers and Scott (1975) that the first few readings with the NCT are often a little higher, by about 1 mmHg, than subsequent readings. This he attributes to an apprehension factor. The NCT does not, however, show the gradual decrease in intraocular pressure with repeated measures as shown by the Goldmann instrument (Moses and Liu, 1968; Krakau and Wilke, 1971).

The ease with which tonometric measurements can be made with this instrument has made the routine measurement of intraocular pressure a much more viable proposition to the optometrist. In addition to this, it is particularly valuable in children and in people who cannot tolerate objects touching the eye (Sorensen, 1975). Whether these advantages outweigh the disadvantages of high cost and of complexity, which with time is bound to cause maintenance problems, is difficult to decide. There is little doubt, however, that it is a pioneering instrument in the measurement of intraocular pressure.

References

BURMAN, B. (1974). Comparison between the NCT and Mackay–Marg tonometer. *American Journal of Optometry and Physiological Optics*, **51**, 34

DUKE-ELDER, S. (1952). The phasic variations in ocular tension in primary glaucoma. *American Journal of Ophthalmology*, **35**, 1

DUNN, J. S. and BRUBAKER, R. F. (1973). Perkins applanation tonometer. *Archives of Opthalmology*, **89**, 149

FORBES, M., PICO, G. and GROLMAN, B. (1974). A non contact applanation tonometer: Description and clinical evaluation. *Archives of Ophthalmology*, **91**, 134

FRIEDENWALD, J. S. (1957). Tonometer calibration. *Transactions of the American Academy of Ophthalmology and Otolaryngology*, **61**, 108

GLOSTER, J. (1965). Tonometry and tonography. *International Ophthalmology Clinics*, **5**, 911

GLOSTER, J. and MARTIN, B. (1965). Evaluation of the Posner–Inglima Applanometer. *British Journal of Ophthalmology*, **49**, 617

GROLMAN, B. (1972). A new tonometer system. *American Journal of Optometry and Archives of the American Academy of Optometry*, **49**, 646

HILTON, G. F. and SHAFFER, R. N. (1966). Electronic applanation tonometry. *American Journal of Ophthalmology*, **62**, 838

HORIE, T. and KITAZAWA, Y. (1979). The clinical significance of diurnal pressure variation in primary open-angle glaucoma. *Japanese Journal of Ophthalmology*, **23**, 310

JAIN, M. R. and MARMION, V. J. (1976a). Rapid pneumatic and Mackay–Marg applanation tonometry to evaluate the postural effects on intraocular pressure. *British Journal of Ophthalmology*, **60**, 687

JAIN, M. R. and MARMION, V. J. (1976b). A clinical evaluation of the applanation Pneuma-tonograph. *British Journal of Ophthalmology*, **60**, 107

KITAZAWA, Y. and HORIE, T. (1975). Diurnal variation in intraocular pressure in primary open-angle glaucoma. *American Journal of Ophthalmology*, **79**, 557

KOESTER, C. J., CAMPBELL, C. J. and DUNN, A. (1980). Ophthalmic optical instruments: Two recent developments. *Japanese Journal of Ophthalmology*, **24**, 1

KRAKAU, C. E. T. and WILKE, K. (1971). On repeated tonometry. *Acta Ophthalmologica*, **49**, 611

MOSES, R. A. (1958). The Goldmann applanation tonometer. *American Journal of Ophthalmology*, **46**, 865

MOSES, R. A. (1975). Intraocular pressure. In *Adler's Physiology of the Eye: Clinical Application*, 6th Edn., p. 179. Edited by R. A. Moses. Mosby, St. Louis

MOSES, R. A. and GRODZKI, W. J. (1979). The Pneumatonograph: A laboratory study. *Archives of Ophthalmology*, **97**, 547

MOSES, R. A. and LIU, C. H. (1968). Repeated applanation tonometry. *American Journal of Ophthalmology*, **66**, 89

MOSES, R. A., MARG, E. and OECHSLI, R. (1962). Evaluation of the basic validity and clinical usefulness of the Mackay–Marg tonometer. *Investigative Ophthalmology*, **1**, 78

MYERS, K. J. and SCOTT, C. A. (1975). The non contact tonometer: Variability and corneal staining. *American Journal of Optometry and Physiological Optics*, **52**, 36

PERKINS, E. S. (1965). Hand-held applanation tonometry. *British Journal of Ophthalmology*, **49**, 469

POSNER, A. and INGLIMA, R. (1962a). Methods used in recalibration of Maklakov tonometer. *Eye, Ear, Nose and Throat Monthly*, **41**, 1028

POSNER, A. and INGLIMA, R. (1962b). Modified conversion tables for the Maklakov tonometer. *Eye, Ear, Nose and Throat Monthly*, **41**, 638

POSNER, A. and INGLIMA, R. (1968). Evaluation of the Tonair tonometer versus Schiotz tonometer and Applanometer. *Eye, Ear, Nose and Throat Monthly*, **47**, 469

QUIGLEY, H. A. and LANGHAM, M. E. (1975). Comparative intraocular pressure measurements with the Pneumatonograph and Goldmann tonometer. *American Journal of Opthalmology*, **80**, 266

ROSENTHAL, J. and WERNER, D. L. (1969). *Tonometry and Glaucoma Detection*. The Professional Press, Chicago

SORENSEN, P. N. (1975). The non contact tonometer: Clinical evaluation on normal and diseased eyes. *Acta Ophthalmologica*, **53**, 513

STEINBERG, P. M. (1965). The Tonair applanation tonometer – a clinical evaluation. *Optical Journal and Review of Optometry*, **102**, 33

STEINBERG, P. M. and ADISE, H. H. (1964). The Steinberg–Adise air tonometer: An introductory report. *Optical Journal and Review of Optometry*, **101**, 25

TIERNEY, J. P. and RUBIN, M. L. (1966). A clinical evaluation of the electronic applanation tonometer. *American Journal of Ophthalmology*, **62**, 263

WALLACE, J. and LOVELL, H. G. (1968). Perkins hand-held applanation tonometer: A clinical evaluation. *British Journal of Ophthalmology*, **52**, 568

WHITTY, H. P. B. (1969). Trial results of a hand-held applanation apparatus. *British Journal of Ophthalmology*, **53**, 664

4

Field equipment

The visual field has been defined by Tate and Lynn (1977) as all the space that one eye can see at any given instant in time. It is normally measured in degrees from the line of sight and on average extends, when a patient is looking straight ahead, 65 degrees upwards, 75 degrees downwards, 60 degrees inwards (towards the nose) and 95 degrees outwards (temporally) (*see Figure 4.1*).

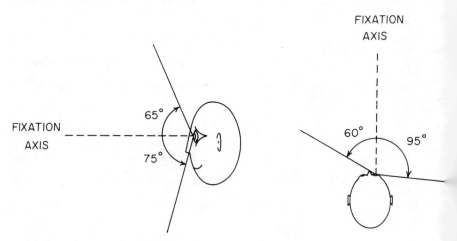

Figure 4.1. The normal extent of the visual field

Within the area of the visual field the sensitivity of the eye, which is defined as the inverse of the threshold, varies according to certain parameters, such as adaptation level and target colour, size and exposure time. At normal room illumination the eye is most sensitive at the fovea, i.e. along the line of sight. In the dark, the eye's most sensitive area shifts to a region 10–30 degrees away from the fovea (*see Figure 4.2*). Visual field examinations are normally undertaken in the lower photopic ranges at which the fovea is most sensitive.

Certain types of ocular pathology can result in defects of the visual field. These can take the form of isolated areas of depressed sensitivity, known as scotoma, or reductions in the overall size of the visual field. Depending upon the type and stage of the pathology, these two defects can occur independently of each other or in combination. An understanding of the exact nature of the defects that occur as a result of a specific pathology is important when different techniques of visual field examination are considered and when particular pieces of visual field equipment are

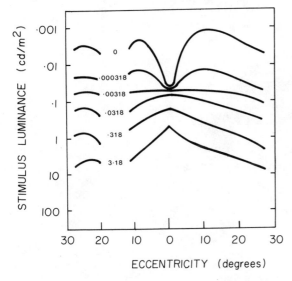

Figure 4.2. Profile field plots at six different background luminance levels. The numbers on each curve are the background luminance levels in candela/m². After Greve (1973)

assessed. The next two sections of this chapter therefore contain brief descriptions of the types of defects that arise from the more frequently encountered ocular pathologies.

Glaucoma

By far the most common reason for an optometrist to conduct a visual field examination is the suspicion of open-angle glaucoma. This condition is characterized by an increase in intraocular pressure which results in damage to the fibres at the optic nerve head. The exact reason as to why these fibres should be damaged prior to any others is still not fully understood. It is this damage, however, which causes the visual field defects and optic nerve head cupping which are pathognomonic of glaucoma. The most frequent field defects found in early cases of open-angled glaucoma are small, isolated scotoma in the central 30 degrees (Aulhorn and Harms, 1967; Armaly, 1971). Peripheral nasal steps and concentric contraction are found less frequently. If the condition of glaucoma is allowed to advance, then these defects enlarge and connect to the blind spot, and so form large arcuate defects. Aulhorn and Karmeyer (1976) have investigated the frequency with which early scotoma occur in specific regions of the visual field. It can be seen from their data (*Figure 4.3*) that early defects most often occur in the inferior nasal region within

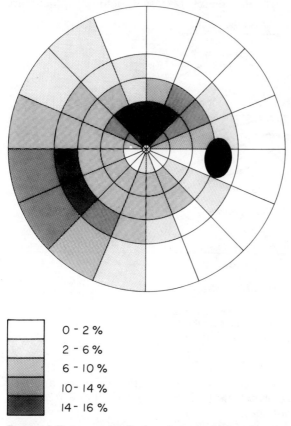

	0 - 2 %
	2 - 6 %
	6 - 10 %
	10 - 14 %
	14 - 16 %

Figure 4.3. Frequency distribution of scotoma in glaucomatous patients with early visual field defects. After Aulhorn and Karmeyer (1976)

an arc of about 10 to 30 degrees from the fovea, and just superior to the macula. However, the important point to notice, as far as the design of field equipment goes, is that these isolated, small scotoma can occur almost anywhere within the central region of the visual field.

Other pathologies

While there are many other pathologies that result in visual field defects, the frequency with which a visual field examination is conducted in order to assist in the diagnosis of one of these conditions is rare in comparison with glaucoma. The reason for this is threefold. First, the incidence of these pathologies is much lower than that of glaucoma. Second, these pathologies often give rise to specific symptoms or are related to other pathological conditions that result in the patient being referred directly to the ophthalmologist or neurologist without first being seen by an optometrist. Third, the other signs or symptoms of the pathology may be sufficient to allow the optometrist to confidently refer without the need of a field examination. Having said this, it is still important that the defects associated with the pathologies listed below should be detectable with the field equipment found in an optometric practice.

1. Diseases that affect the visual pathways. These conditions give rise to sector shaped defects which usually occur over large areas of the visual field and may, in the early stages of the condition, be very shallow;
2. Toxic amblyopias. The majority cause central scotoma although some, notably quinine, may cause peripheral field loss;
3. Optic nerve lesions. Retro-bulbar neuritis and papillitis cause small, deep, central scotoma, while papilloedema causes an enlargement of the blind spot.
4. Retinal lesions. Retinitis pigmentosa often causes a ring scotoma and a gradual loss of the peripheral field. Arterial occulsions cause deep scotoma which correspond to the area of retina supplied by the occluded artery, while venous occlusions create field losses due to the existence of blood that occludes the visual cells. Retinal detachments cause isolated defects that correspond to the area of the detachment.

An excellent and more detailed description of the field defects associated with specific pathologies can be found in Reed and Drance (1972).

Techniques of visual field examination

In order to test the visual field, the clinician needs to be able to present targets or stimuli in different parts of the field and ascertain whether or not the patient can see them. There are two basic ways in which this can be done. One is known as the kinetic technique while the other is known as the static technique.

In the kinetic technique, the clinician uses a target of constant intensity and gradually moves it from the periphery of the field, where it cannot be seen, towards the fovea. The point at which the target is first seen is recorded as the limit of the field of view or threshold for that stimulus. It is known as the kinetic technique because the target moves. In order to detect a scotoma within the threshold region the clinician continues to move the target towards the fovea, the patient having been instructed to report if the target fades or disappears. By using the same kinetic stimulus along a whole series of meridians, a ring of points can be plotted which, when joined by a line, is known as an isopter. Isopters in the central 30 degrees are approximately circular. By using targets of different intensities, a series of isopters can be plotted which will fall at varying distances from the fovea. When drawn together, the appearance is not unlike that of contour lines on a relief map (*see Figure 4.4*).

With the static technique, the clinician keeps the position of the stimulus constant and increases its intensity until it is detected. The recorded threshold is the lowest intensity of the stimulus that can be reliably detected by the patient. It is known as the static technique because the target remains stationary. The likelihood of detecting scotoma with the static technique is dependent upon the number of points tested.

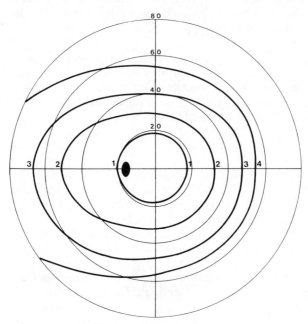

Figure 4.4. Field plot of four isopters

The distinction between the kinetic and static technique is represented on the profile field diagram shown in *Figure 4.5*. Kinetic perimetry can be thought of as moving targets horizontally across this diagram, while static techniques can be thought of as moving targets vertically.

When kinetic perimetry is used as a screening procedure, the technique adopted varies from perimetrist to perimetrist. Some will use a whole series of targets and plot each isopter. Others may not plot an isopter at all, but simply search for scotoma in highly suspect areas. Because of the variety of ways in which kinetic perimetry can be performed and because many perimetrists do not fully define their methods (e.g. area of field covered, speed of stimulus movement), different perimetrists claim different sensitivities for what appear to be the same technique; sensitivity here is defined as the ability to detect a scotoma. The more sensitive a technique is the greater will be the percentage of scotoma that it detects.

In the early days of perimetry, kinetic techniques were used almost exclusively because the technique of static perimetry with the then available equipment was either impossible or exceedingly laborious. Just imagine having to go through 70 or 80 points in the visual field and independently determine the threshold at each one. The almost exclusive use of kinetic techniques has led to a classification of field defects with isopter diagrams. A quick examination of the classic text by Harrington (1956) on the visual field will reveal just how entrenched the current understanding of field defects are with isopter diagrams.

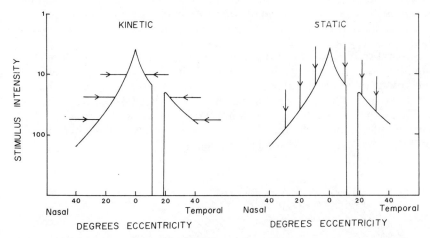

Figure 4.5. Kinetic perimetry is represented on the left of the figure by the horizontal arrows. Static perimetry is represented on the right by the vertical arrows

The main problem of static perimetry, namely the time taken to perform an adequate field examination, has been overcome, to a large extent, by the adoption of two modifications to the way in which static perimetry is performed.

In the first of these, the stimuli are initially presented at what is calculated to be a slightly supra threshold intensity. If the patient detects this stimulus then no further testing at that location is conducted, it being assumed that a scotoma does not exist. If the target is not seen then its intensity can be increased in order to establish the threshold and hence the depth of the scotoma. Because of the way stimuli are presented, the technique is often referred to as the supra threshold static technique. It should be pointed out that while it is ideal for detecting fairly deep scotoma, it is not suitable for detecting shallow scotoma or slight differences between the fields of the two eyes. The technique is, however, particularly suitable for glaucoma screening where the most common type of defect is a small, fairly deep scotoma within the central 30 degrees.

The second modification to the static technique involves the simultaneous presentation of more than one supra threshold stimulus. The technique is known as multiple-stimulus static perimetry for obvious reasons. With this technique, the patient reports the number of stimuli seen which is usually made to vary between each presentation. In addition to quickening the field examination, the multiple-stimulus technique operates in a relatively fail-safe manner when the patient's attention lapses. When the perimetrist investigates the region within a target's isopter with kinetic perimetry (i.e. when looking for isolated field defects) any loss of attention by the patient is interpreted by the perimetrist as indicating that no field defect exists because the patient neglects to report that the target has disappeared. With the multiple-stimulus static technique this is not the case. The patient has to report the number of stimuli seen, and any lapse of attention or guessing would result in the patient reporting either no targets seen or an incorrect number seen (75% chance; multiple-stimulus static perimetry normally presents up to four stimuli at a time). As a result, the perimetrist would check the response with a second presentation.

Several researchers have reported that with either one or both of these modifications, the static technique of visual field examination is superior to the kinetic one in being able to detect the small, isolated scotoma that are often the first and only sign of glaucomatous damage (Aulhorn and Harms, 1972; Drance, Wheeler and Patullo, 1967; Greve and Verduin, 1976). Hence, the static technique has, over the last few years, become the preferred technique of visual field screening.

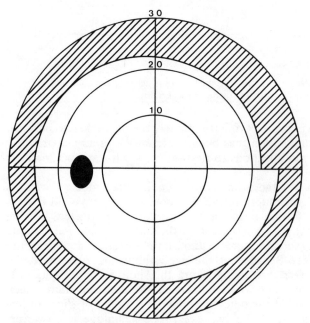

Figure 4.6. A single isopter that demonstrates nasal step. The heavily shaded area is the blind spot

One of the early types of field defect seen in open-angled glaucoma is called a nasal step. It is an isopter anomaly caused by the sensitivity above the horizontal meridian being different to that below, in the nasal field (*see Figure 4.6*). Because this sensitivity difference may, in the early stages of glaucoma, be only slight it is more easily detected with the kinetic technique. Several perimetrists have, thus, recently advocated a glaucoma screening technique that combines both static and kinetic techniques. One such routine is known as the Armaly–Drance technique (Rock, Drance and Morgan, 1973) which includes 72 supra threshold static presentations and eight kinetic measurements of the nasal isopter above and below the horizontal meridian. While this technique is not without criticisms (Greve and Verduin, 1976) it is generally accepted as an excellent technique of visual screening for glaucoma.

Other researchers have based glaucoma screening techniques solely on static perimetry and claim as high, if not higher, sensitivities than the Armaly–Drance technique. Comparisons of different techniques are, however, very difficult to make due to inhomogeneities of population groups and different definitions as to what constitutes a glaucomatous field defect. Since the advent of the current generation of perimeters, however, no researcher has advocated a glaucoma screening programme based solely upon kinetic techniques. In a recent comparison of visual field screening techniques in which a kinetic technique was compared with several other techniques, the solely kinetic one was only 32 per cent sensitive (i.e. was only capable of detecting 32 out of 100 cases in which a field defect existed), while the more elaborate static technique detected 100 per cent (Greve and Verduin, 1976).

Standardization of field equipment

The International Perimetric Society has recently produced some recommended standards for perimetry (International Peritric Society, 1976). These standards have been specifically written for the benefit of the practitioner. They currently take the form of a series of recommendations as to which parameters should be specified in a testing situation and the manner in which these parameters should be specified. They have not, as yet, recommended specific parameter values because at the present time the optimal conditions for a field examination are still unknown.

Their major recommendations are as follows:

1. Photometric standards, such as the background intensity and the target intensity, should be expressed in luminance units measured at the entrance pupil of the eye being tested;
2. Coloured targets should be specified by the wavelength composition of the stimulus reaching the eye;
3. Test target parameters (size, configuration and exposure duration or rate of translation), viewing distance and location of the target within the visual field should be specified.

These recommendations are very important because they allow the visual stimulus to be defined. The provision of levels of chart illumination, such as that often provided with the tanget screen (7 ft candles), are not recommended because they take no account of the reflective properties of the screen and therefore do not fully define the visual stimulus.

The working group feel that it is the responsibility of the instrument manufacturer to provide the clinician with equipment and calibration devices capable of meeting their recommendations. While very few pieces of field equipment currently meet these recommendations, it is hoped that future designs will.

Evaluation of a piece of field equipment

There are three ways in which a piece of field equipment can be evaluated:

1. The technical specifications of the instrument can be examined to see whether it is capable of meeting the Interprofessional Standards Committees recommendations (*see* previous section). These recommendations allow the perimetrist to define *fully* the testing conditions and therefore allow other perimetrists to repeat the measurements under identical conditions;
2. The technical specifications can be examined in the light of our current understanding of ocular pathology to see whether the instrument is capable of presenting optimal stimuli for the detection of defects. For example, we can see whether the instrument can present stimuli in those regions of the field where defects most often occur. Similarly, we can observe what the stimulus intensity steps are in order to establish whether it is capable of detecting shallow scotoma. Other examples relate to the size and colour of stimuli, whether provision is made for corrections to be worn and whether the instrument can perform static perimetry.
3. The final and possibly the most valuable way of evaluating a piece of field equipment is to look at its clinical sensitivity and specificity. Sensitivity in this context is defined as its ability to detect defects when they are present, e.g. a piece of field equipment can be said to be 95 per cent sensitive if it can detect 95 out of 100 cases with a defect. Specificity is a measure of how many cases that do *not* have a defect are reported as having one by a piece of equipment, i.e. the number of false positives.

To say a piece of equipment is very specific (i.e. it never fails a patient who does not have a defect) is of little value without also saying how sensitive the piece of equipment is. Similarly, to say that a piece of equipment can detect 100 per cent of cases with a defect is of little value without a measure of how specific it is. Equipment can always be made more sensitive, but this invariably results in the equipment being less specific and visa versa.

In a discussion of individual pieces of field equipment it is not always possible to give data concerning its sensitivity and specificity. The reasons for this are two-fold. First, many pieces of equipment can be used in a variety of ways and the equipment's ability to detect a defect is dependent upon the way it is used. For example, someone who spends half-an-hour carefully measuring the visual field of a subject is going to find more defects than someone who spends 10 min, even though they use the same piece of equipment. Second, the definition as to whether a defect exists or not is usually based upon the measurements taken with another piece of field equipment or field measuring technique, which itself will only have a certain sensitivity. Evaluations of a piece of equipment or a technique of measuring the visual field are, therefore, really comparisons of equipment or techniques.

In the following discussions about individual pieces of field equipment, all three types of evaluation are given whenever possible. However, due to the problems of measurement of sensitivity and specificity, mentioned above, the majority of evaluations are based solely upon technical specifications.

Introduction to the instruments

To aid the following discussions, visual vield equipment has been divided into four main categories; tangent screens, arc and bowl perimeters, screeners and computerized equipment.

Tangent screens

Tangent screens use a flat surface to test the visual field. The screen can be attached to a wall or it can come as part of a piece of equipment. Tangent screen instruments only allow the central 30 degrees or so of the visual field to be tested.

Arc and bowl perimeters

Arc and bowl perimeters allow the perimetrist to examine both the central and peripheral field. Because the targets are usually presented closer to the patient's eye than with tangent screens, these instruments do not normally offer the same degree of precision within the central field.

Screeners

While almost any piece of field equipment can be used to screen quickly the visual field for defects, some pieces of equipment have been specifically designed for this purpose. It is this latter group that will be discussed under this heading.

Computerized equipment

Computerized equipment will be discussed separately, although, in effect, each piece of computerized field equipment could fit into one of the previous three groups.

Tangent screens

Bjerrum screen

The Bjerrum screen is a black cloth fixed against the wall at 1 m from the patient (2 m versions are occasionally found and are more accurate for charting scotoma). Black thread is sewn onto the cloth to give a series of radial and circumferential lines as shown in *Figure 4.7*. These lines are normally invisible to the patient, but can be seen by the optometrist and are used to determine the position of the target during the test. A white spot is attached to the centre of the screen which provides a fixation point for the patient.

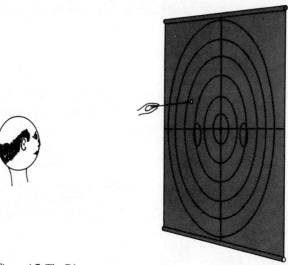

Figure 4.7. The Bjerrum screen

In use, one of a series of targets of different size and colour is attached to the end of a black wand which is held by the perimetrist. Because both the wand and the screen are black the wand remains invisible to the patient as long as fixation is maintained at the centre of the screen. The perimetrist moves the target in from the periphery of the field, just in front of the plane of the screen, until the subject just notices it. Scotoma within the area of a target's isopter are detected by continuing to move the spot towards the fixation point and asking the patient to report if, at any time, it disappears. Black pins can be placed into the cloth at the positions where the target appears or disappears. At the end of the test, the positions of these pins are recorded onto special chart paper which can be kept with the patient's record. To test the patient's response within the area of a target's isopter, the wand can be rapidly twirled by the perimetrist to expose the reverse side of the target, which is usually painted black. If the patient is attentive during this procedure then he or she should report that the target has disappeared. To test the patient's response in this way is very important because the twirling can be made to closely simulate a small, deep scotoma similar to that found in glaucoma. If the patient immediately recognizes that the target has disappeared, then the perimetrist can have some confidence in the test's ability to detect this type of defect. On the other hand, if the patient fails to recognize that the target has disappeared until verbally cued by the perimetrist, then little faith can be put in the test's ability to detect early glaucomatous defects.

The two main advantages of the Bjerrum screen are that it is cheap and versatile. It is possible to use targets of almost any size or colour, to set the background intensity at any level and to move the targets in any direction along any meridian at whatever speed the perimetrist believes optimal.

The main disadvantages of the Bjerrum screen are:

1. It contains no calibration facilities and therefore does not fulfil the recommendations of the Interprofessional Standards of Visual Field Testing Committee (International Perimetric Society, 1976);
2. The targets quickly get damaged and soiled;
3. It cannot be used to perform static perimetry, which is currently believed to be the best technique for detecting the isolated defects that are commonly found in early glaucoma;
4. The size of the targets make the instrument insensitive to defects within the central 25 degrees. The smallest target normally available with the Bjerrum screen is a 1/1000 W. This target produces a roughly circular isopter at about 25 degrees from the fovea (Harrington, 1956). As the sensitivity of the eye increases within this region, so too must the depth of any detectable defect (Henson, 1980).

This fourth point is explained in more detail in *Figure 4.8* where the position of the 1/1000 W target has been marked on a profile field plot. It can be seen from this figure that while the target is at threshold at about 25

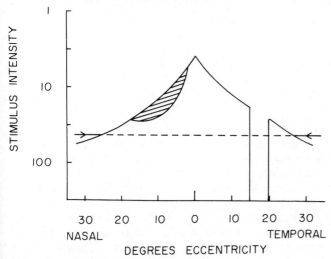

Figure 4.8. The shaded area represents the type of scotoma that would be missed with a 1/1000 W target on a Bjerrum screen

degrees from the fovea (the position of the 1/1000 W isopter), it represents a supra threshold target within this area, which is, at the fovea, approximately 1 log unit above threshold. It may very well be impossible to detect shallow defects within this region of the visual field, which is, according to Aulhorn and Karmeyer (1976), the area where most glaucoma defects first occur.

Juler scotometer

The Juler Scotometer projects a small spot of light onto a grey 1 m tangent screen (*see Figure 4.9*). It is usually bought as an accessory to the Fincham–Sutcliffe screener (*see* pp. 74–76), but can, in fact, be used on any grey screen. The scotometer is held behind the patient so that the patient is unaware of the direction in which it points. The diameter of the projected spot can be varied from 1 to 30 mm in discrete steps and can be coloured red, green or white. The instrument is exceedingly versatile and

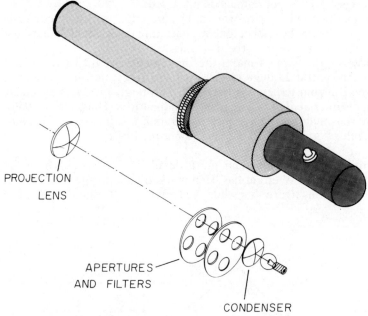

PROJECTION
LENS

APERTURES
AND FILTERS

CONDENSER

Figure 4.9. The Juler scotometer

yet simple. It is an improvement over the standard Bjerrum screen as it requires neither a wand nor a perimetrist to stand in the field of view. The manufacturers (Keeler) recommend that the instrument be held in one hand while the field is charted with the other. The weight of the instrument is a little excessive for this to be done with ease. It is, however, possible to have it mounted on a small stand, which overcomes this problem.

The instrument has a small button attached to it which enables the perimetrist to silently extinguish the light. This type of attachment is exceedingly useful in practice as it allows the perimetrist to check the patient's response. If several checks are made during the course of the examination, the perimetrist can gauge how reliable the patient is and ascertain what degree of confidence he can apply to the results.

The instrument has the following major shortcomings:

1. It does not include any calibration facilities;
2. There is no built-in control over the background illumination;
3. It cannot be used for static perimetry because the operator cannot accurately position the stimulus when the projector light is off.

The last problem has been overcome by Hagedoorn and Van Den Bosch (1955) with the development of a double-projection campimeter. This instrument, which is considerably more sophisticated than the Juler scotometer, projects a second spot onto a field chart in a position that corresponds with the stimulus on the screen. To perform static perimetry with this instrument, the perimetrist first positions the spot on the field chart and then triggers the shutter, which exposes the stimulus to the patient in the corresponding position on the screen. In addition to the automatic shutter, the instrument has a much larger range of neutral density (ND) filters. The instrument has been reviewed by Greve (1973) who feels that it is superior to the Goldmann instrument for evaluating the central fields by either static or kinetic techniques.

Bausch and Lomb Autoplot

The Autoplot is a projection instrument for use on a 1 m grey tangent screen. The instrument has a pen stylus which is moved over an illuminated panel upon which is placed a field chart. The pen is connected via a pantograph device to a vertically mounted projector which places a spot on the screen at the same relative position as the pen on the chart (*see Figure 4.10*). The patient, whose head is stabilized with a chin rest, looks over the

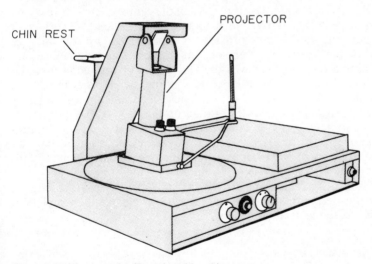

Figure 4.10. The Autoplot (Bausch and Lomb)

top of the projector. The diameter of the spot can be varied from 0.5 mm to 15 mm in seven discrete steps and can be coloured red, green, blue or white. Unfortunately, the instrument cannot control the intensity of the stimulus, although the contrast of the spot can be changed by varying the background illumination on the screen.

This instrument overcomes many of the problems related to the Bjerrum screen and is considerably neater and more convenient to use than either the Juler scotometer or the double-projection campimeter. Its lack of screen and stimulus calibration facilities and its inability to perform static perimetry are disappointing.

In a recent paper by Schoessler and Uniacke (1977) some modifications to the Autoplot have been described that allow the instrument to be standardized to the Goldmann perimeter. One of the modifications is to replace the coloured filters with a neutral density wedge such that the intensity of the target can be varied. With this and with one or two other relatively minor modifications, such as the incorporation of a light meter and a shutter for static perimetry, the Autoplot could become an excellent piece of field measuring equipment.

Inami Opto-campimeter

This instrument is similar to the Bausch and Lomb Autoplot, but has the additional facility that it allows flicker perimetry.

Arc and bowl perimeters

The arc perimeter

The arc perimeter is a very simple instrument composed of a semi-circular arc, the inside surface of which is painted matt black. The patient's head is fixed such that the eye under test is located at the centre of curvature of the arc. The visual field is tested by moving a target along the black surface of the perimeter until the patient just sees it. The targets are the same as those used for the Bjerrum screen, i.e. small discs of varying colour and size attached to the end of black wands. The arc can be rotated around the fixation point, which is located at the centre of the arc, in order to test the visual field along any meridian. The position of the wand and the angle of the arc can be read off from scales printed on the back of the perimeter.

Some arc perimeters have a light attached to them that evenly illuminates the whole of the perimeter arc. The provision of this type of background illuminator is particularly valuable due to the difficulty, with normal overhead lighting, of evenly illuminating a 180 degree arc. This instrument suffers from the same disadvantages as the Bjerrum screen, but does allow the perimetrist to measure the full extent of the visual field rather than just the central 30 degrees.

Aimark projection perimeter

The Aimark projection perimeter is an instrument that replaces the wand and disc targets of the arc perimeter with a projection device. (*see Figure 4.11*). The inside surface of the arc is painted a grey colour so that the projected target can be seen. The colour and size of the target can be selected via a range of filters and apertures fixed within the projector. The spot of light on the screen is moved by rotation of a knob that is attached, via a cable, to a mirror that reflects the projected light onto the arc. The knob also moves a pin point across a field chart, the position of which corresponds to the position of the spot of light on the arc. This pin point can be pushed into the chart when a patient first sees the target and, at the end of the examination, the pin pricks can be joined together to produce an isopter. The Aimark perimeter has no built-in background illuminator and does not contain any calibration facilities for either the stimulus or background.

The value of both the arc perimeter and the Aimark projection perimeter is limited to establishing the total extent of the visual field by

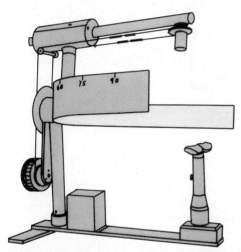

Figure 4.11. The Aimark projection arc perimeter (Clement Clarke)

kinetic techniques and whether any contraction has occurred. These instruments are not sensitive enough to be used for the detection of early glaucomatous damage that occurs within the central 30 degrees.

The Goldmann perimeter

The Goldmann instrument is a bowl perimeter, the inside radius of which is 30 cm. Stimuli are projected onto the inside surface of the bowl, which is sprayed an off-white colour and has a coefficient of reflectance of 0.7. The stimuli are moved via a pantographic arrangement which connects the projector to the stylus of the operator's pen (*see Figure 4.12*). The pantographic arrangement allows the position of the stimulus within the patient's visual field to correspond with the position of the stylus on the field chart.

The intensity and size of the projected stimulus is controlled via a series of three ND filters (0.5, 1.0 and 1.5 log units) and six apertures (*see Table 4.1*). The maximum intensity of the stimulus, i.e. with no ND filters in the light path, is set at 1000 asb (318 cd/m^2) with the aid of an internal luxmeter and rheostat. The three ND filters reduce this intensity to 315 asb (100 cd/m^2), 100 asb (31.8 cd/m^2) and 31.5 asb (10 cd/m^2), respectively. Goldmann selected the target size steps and the intensity steps such that, under the conditions of his perimeter, they would be equivalent. Increasing the size of the target by one step would have the same effect as increasing target luminance by one step (0.5 log units). Unfortunately, the laws that

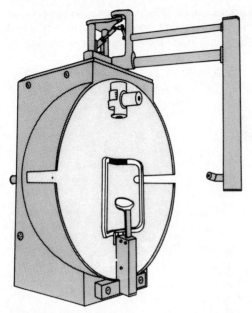

Figure 4.12. The Goldmann bowl perimeter (Haag–Streit)

relate to spatial summation upon which Goldmann based his calculations show a considerable amount of individual variability. Thus, the relationship between these two parameters is frequently found to differ from that calculated by Goldmann (Greve, 1973).

TABLE 4.1. The size and angular subtense of the Goldmann targets (long axis, *see* Greve, 1973)*

Goldmann size	0	I	II	III	IV	V
Nominal size	0.0625	0.25	1.0	4.0	16.0	64.0
Angular subtence (min of arc)	3.78	7.68	15.36	30.71	61.30	122.56

*Because of the nature of the projector, the targets appear elliptical upon the bowl surface

The background luminance of the bowl is controlled via a variable aperture and is normally set at 31.5 asb ($10\,cd/m^2$) by visually matching its intensity with that of the calibrated light source. It can, however, be reduced to values much lower than this, if desired. Attached to the back of the bowl is a telescope through which the perimetrist can view the patient's eye. This telescope allows the perimetrist to check that the patient maintains fixation throughout the field examination.

The short working distance and small target sizes of the Goldmann instrument mean that accurate refractions with near additions (if necessary) must be worn while testing the central field. Failure to do this can result in large errors with the smaller targets (Sloan, 1961). A lens holder is provided with the instrument to make this possible in patients who do not have an adequate prescription for a 30 cm working distance.

The Goldmann perimeter was originally designed for kinetic perimetry. It has, however, been modified for static perimetry by the addition of a further four ND filters which allow the target luminance to be controlled in 0.1 log unit steps from 0 to 1.9 log units. This range can be increased by the addition of filter caps over the end of the projector. In addition to this, an attachment to the pantograph can be added that aids profile perimetry. Even with these modifications, the Goldmann perimeter is not ideally suited for static perimetry. In the first case, it does not allow exposure times to be controlled with any precision because of the lack of automatic shutters. Second, the stability of the pantographic arrangement and the size of the charts mean that precise location of the target within the cupula is difficult (Greve, 1973) and finally, the elaborate procedure necessary for static perimetry is time consuming.

The Goldmann instrument, however, is one of the most widely used perimeters in ophthalmology. Its precise control over most stimulus parameters, such as background and stimulus intensities, and its ability to perform both static and kinetic perimetry over the whole of the visual field, has made it an ideal choice for many ophthalmalogical clinics. In optometry, where glaucoma screening is the main requirement of a perimeter, it has not found such a wide acceptance due to its high cost and its protracted examination procedures.

Inami, Topcon and Takagi projection perimeters

These three perimeters have identical stimulus specifications to that of the Goldmann instrument and almost identical constructions. Two of them, Topcon and Takagi, offer an additional attachment that allows them to perform flicker perimetry.

The Tubinger perimeter (Oculus)

The Tubinger perimeter (*see Figure 4.13*) is one of the most sophisticated bowl perimeters. In addition to static and kinetic perimetry, it can monitor the dark adaptation process, measure peripheral visual acuity and investigate the critical fusion frequency.

Targets are projected onto the inside surface of the bowl (radius 33 cm) which is painted matt white and has a coefficient of reflectance of 0.8. The background intensity, for which calibration facilities are provided, is normally set at 10 asb ($3.18 \, cd/m^2$), but can be adjusted, with ND filters and an occluder, to any value between 10 and 0 asb. The stimuli, for which calibration facilities are provided, can be varied over an 8 log unit range with a series of two ND filter wheels, the maximum intensity being 1000 asb. In addition to this, there are eight different sizes of stimuli, all expressed in the min of arc they subtend at the eye (7, 10, 12, 18, 27, 44, 69 and 116 min of arc). The exposure time of the target is controlled via an electromagnetic shutter that allows stimulus presentation times of 0.1 to 1 s.

The Tubinger instrument allows, within the central 30 degrees, much greater cartographic accuracy than does the Goldmann instrument. This is achieved by two separate modes of operation. In the first mode, which is similar to that of the Goldmann, the visual field chart covers the whole 180 degrees of the bowl, while in the second one, the same degree of stylus movement covers only the central 30 degrees of the field. The two types of test charts used are shown in *Figure 4.14*.

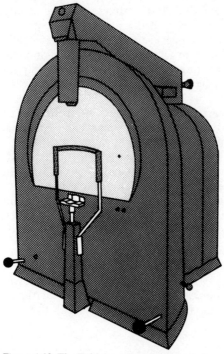

Figure 4.13. The Tubinger perimeter (Oculus)

The Tubinger perimeter is primarily designed for static profile perimetry along different meridians of the eye. The meridian along which the measurements are to be taken is selected by rotating the whole projector mechanism around the instrument's anterioposterior axis, which coincides with the patient's line of sight. The target can then be moved to different positions along this meridian via the turning of a knob attached to the back of the instrument. This arrangement allows the target to be positioned within the bowl with far greater precision than in the Goldmann instrument. The disadvantage of this arrangement is that kinetic perimetry can only practically be performed with the target moving meridionally. This restriction makes the plotting of the size of any scotoma or the size of the blind spot exceedingly difficult. It also makes the instrument impractical for the rapid supra threshold static-screening programmes such as that advocated by Rock, Drance and Morgan (1973). The standard fixation point of this instrument, which is adjustable in both size and intensity, can be replaced by four points of light positioned either 2 or 4 degrees from the centre of the bowl. This type of fixation target allows accurate measurements to be made at and close to the fovea.

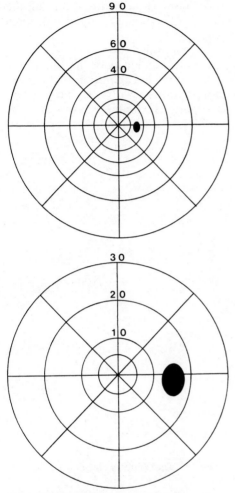

Figure 4.14. The two types of field chart used
with the Tubinger perimeter

The large number of facilities incorporated within this instrument has
made it an ideal instrument for clinical research. Its high expense and
complexity make it less appropriate for routine clinical investigation.

Gambs perimeter

The Gambs perimeter is a hemispheric bowl perimeter of radius 30 cm.
The bowl is made of a transparent material, the inside surface of which is
lined with a matt-white screen and is internally illuminated by a specially
built-in light source. The outside of the bowl carries meridional and isopter
markings which are not visible to the subject through the bowl material
(*see Figure 4.15*). Stimuli are presented via a small hand-held projector
which is placed against the outside of the bowl. The bowl material is such
that it allows the transmission of light from the projector to be seen by the

subject. The operator can mark the positions of an isopter either on the bowl, with a wax pencil, or on a field chart. Fixation is monitored through a small hole in the centre of the bowl.

The intensity of the stimuli can be controlled with five ND filters incorporated within the projector system. The intensity of the stimuli are not specified by the manufacturers and no stimulus calibration facilities are provided. Colour perimetry can be performed with the aid of four non-specified coloured filters also incorporated within the projector. The

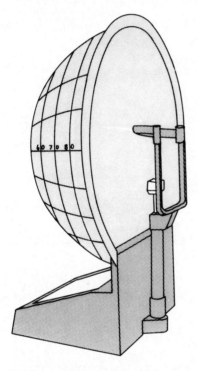

Figure 4.15. The Gambs perimeter

background intensity of the bowl can be adjusted with a diaphragm, the recommended procedure being to visually match its intensity to that of one of the stimuli. While the stimuli are nominally given as the same size as those of the Goldmann, the projection through the lining of the bowl blurrs the target edges to such an extent that they are not strictly equivalent.

The instrument, like the Goldmann, has been primarily designed for kinetic perimetry; it is not possible to control accurately the exposure time of the targets or control the intensity of the target with sufficient precision for static perimetry. It is, however, possible to obtain a projector in which the coloured filters have been replaced by a further set of ND filters. With this projector it is possible to obtain a sufficiently accurate quantitative measure of the sensitivity, as is required for static perimetry.

Rodenstock and Zeiss (Jena) projection perimeters

The Rodenstock instrument offers the same stimulus and background parameters as does the Goldmann instrument, but is constructed in a similar way to the Tubinger instrument. Like the Tubinger instrument it can be operated in <u>two modes,</u> in one of which the chart covers the whole of the visual field and in the other it covers only the central 30 degrees.

The Zeiss (Jena) instrument (*see Figure 4.16*) is also constructed similarly to the Tubinger instrument. The sizes of the stimuli are the same as those on the Goldmann and the instrument has a slightly larger range of

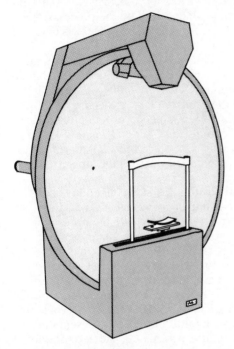

Figure 4.16. The Zeiss bowl perimeter (Zeiss (Jena))

stimulus and background intensities. The maximum stimulus intensity is 1500 asb (rather than 1000) and the maximum background intensity is 50 asb (rather than 31.5 asb). It does not incorporate the facility to expand the charting of the central 30 degrees as does the Rodenstock and Tubinger instruments.

Screeners

Introduction

Many of the recommended techniques of field examination outlined in this chapter, and specified in more detail in texts such as Tate and Lynn (1977), require a considerable amount of time to execute – so much time that they cannot realistically be applied to more than a small percentage of patients. There is a need, especially within the field of optometry, for a more rapid screening technique of field examination that can routinely be applied to large population groups. Visual field screeners have been designed for this purpose.

To understand how screening techniques can quicken the examination, consider that a visual vield examination can actually be divided into two stages: a detection stage and a quantification stage. In the detection stage, the perimetrist searches the visual field for a scotoma, while in the quantification stage he examines the dimensions of a scotoma (its size and its depth). In conventional isopter perimetry, the perimetrist both searches for a scotoma and quantitatively measures its extent. If no defect exists, a lot of time will have been wasted plotting isopters of patients with normal vision. Screening techniques are designed to simply detect scotoma*. By doing away with the quantification stage, they speed up the process of field examination in patients who do not have a defect. If a defect is detected then a quantitative technique is used to measure its extent.

While a screening examination can be conducted with almost any piece of field equipment (e.g. the Armaly–Drance technique with the Goldmann perimeter), some pieces of equipment have been developed specifically for screening. Descriptions of three of these instruments are given below. All three use the multiple-stimulus static technique of examination. Three other screening instruments (the Ocuplot, the Fieldmaster and the Auto Tangent Screen) are discussed in a later section of this chapter under the heading of computerized field equipment. They all use the single-stimulus static technique of field examination.

There is no doubt that the multiple-stimulus static technique has two major advantages over the single-stimulus static technique. First, by presenting more than one stimulus at a time it speeds up the process of the field examination. Second, it operates in a fail-safe manner when the patient's attention lapses. With single-stimulus static techniques there is a tendency for the patient's attention to lapse after the first dozen or so stimulus presentations. This may lead him to continue to respond positively even when a particular stimulus is not seen. This situation would be unlikely to arise with the multiple-stimulus static techniques where the patient has to report the number of stimuli seen in each presentation. If attention lapses and one of the presentations is missed, the patient is more likely to ask the perimetrist to present the stimuli again than to make a guess at the number of stimuli presented. If he or she does choose to guess, the chances of being correct are only 1 in 4, so in the majority of cases a second stimuli presentation would be made.

The Harrington–Flocks screener

The Harrington–Flocks instrument (*see Figure 4.17*) was the first piece of equipment to utilize the multiple-stimulus static technique of visual field investigation. It is designed as a screening instrument only. Once a defect has been detected with this instrument, it is necessary to use another piece of field equipment in order to investigate the depth and extent of the defect.

The instrument consists of a chin rest, an ultraviolet lamp and a series of 20 cards (10 for the right eye and 10 for the left eye) upon each of which is printed a multiple-patterned stimulus in fluorescent sulphide ink. These stimuli are not normally seen when illuminated by white light, but

---

* Some screening instruments are designed to give also some quantitative measures of a defect (e.g. the Friedmann Visual Field Analyser).

fluoresce when illuminated by ultraviolet light. The subjects are instructed to report the number of stimuli (2–4) seen on each card during a single 250 ms flash of ultraviolet light. After each presentation, the perimetrist flips the card forward and down to reveal a new card and a new pattern of stimuli. The size of the stimuli increases towards the periphery of the visual field to take into account the normal changes in retinal sensitivity. The

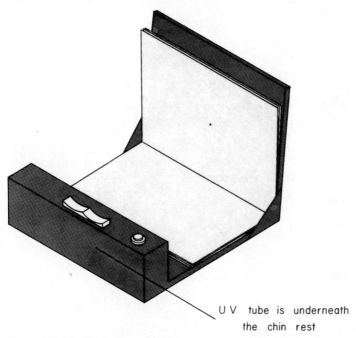

U V tube is underneath
the chin rest

Figure 4.17. The Harrington–Flocks screener (Jenkel–Davidson)

position of the stimuli tested in this screener are shown in *Figure 4.18*. Note that they do not extend beyond 25 degrees from the line of sight.

The main drawbacks of the screener are:

1. There is no means of adjusting the intensity of the stimuli to counteract normal changes in the transparency of the media with age. Thus, in order to avoid a large number of false positives (people with normal fields who fail the test) in elderly patients, the test is made insensitive to relative scotoma in the younger age groups;
2. The cards get soiled after a relatively short period of time to such an extent that the normally invisible targets become visible under white light;
3. An external illuminator is not provided, although Harrington (1956) recommends that the page illumination should be 5 foot candles. 50 LUX.

Numerous clinicians have evaluated the Harrington–Flocks instrument – *see* Harrington and Flocks (1959). Generally, the findings indicate that when a patient fails the test there is a very high probability that a field defect exists, i.e. there are very few false positive responses. No data exists on the number of false negatives, i.e. the number of people with defects who pass this test.

An evaluation of a piece of field equipment cannot be made on just its percentage of false positives or, for that matter, on just its percentage of false negatives. Both these figures must be given. An instrument can always be made more sensitive (less false negatives) or more specific (less

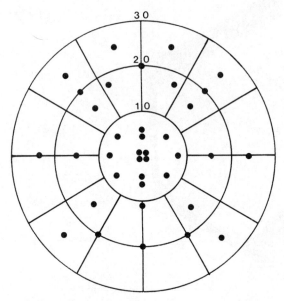

Figure 4.18. The stimulus positions of the Harrington–Flocks screener

false positives) by simple adjusting the intensity of the stimuli. Unfortunately, as you increase the sensitivity of an instrument, you also make it less specific and vice versa.

The Harrington–Flocks instrument has been a pioneer in both field screening and the utilization of the multiple-stimulus technique. Since its design, several other multiple-pattern screeners have been developed which have increased the sensitivity of field screening beyond that available with this instrument.

The Fincham–Sutcliffe screener

The Fincham–Sutcliffe screener (*see Figure 4.19*) is a multiple-stimulus static perimeter designed for use at 1 m, compared with 33 cm for both the Harrington–Flocks and the Visual Field Analyser. The instrument appears as a grey tangent screen behind which are located 67 small, tungsten-filament light sources (*see Figure 4.20*). These light sources, which are presented in a series of 18 patterns, shine through small holes drilled in the tangent screen. In order to account for the normal change in sensitivity

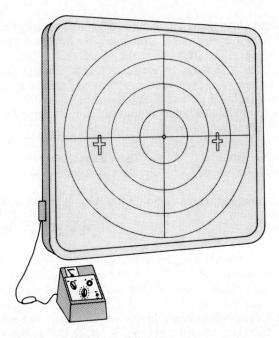

Figure 4.19. The Fincham–Sutcliffe screener (UK Optical)

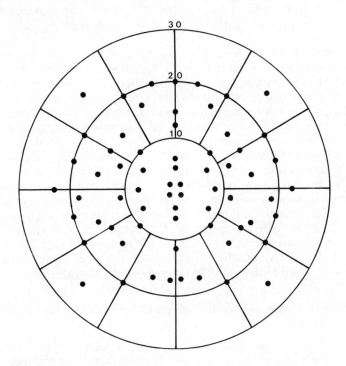

Figure 4.20. The stimulus positions of the Fincham–Sutcliffe screener

across the retina, the holes are increased in size towards the periphery of the field. This allows more light from the bulb to pass through the screen and hence increases the strength of the stimulus.

The instrument contains an electromagnetic shutter that allows the perimetrist to either present each pattern of lights continuously or to present them briefly for periods that vary from 0.1 to 0.9 s. The task of the patient is to report the number of stimuli seen in each of the 18 patterns (the number varies from 2 to 4).

A big advantage of this instrument over the other multiple-pattern screeners is that should any of the targets be missed then a further analysis of it can quickly be made with the Juler projection scotometer (*see* pp. 62-63).

There are, however, three major shortcomings of the instrument:

1. There are no calibration facilities for either the stimuli or the background;
2. There is no built-in background illuminator, although the designers do give fairly detailed instructions on how to install the correct type and give recommended levels of illumination (1–2 lumens/ft^2) (Sutcliffe, 1971);
3. The small tungsten filament lamps give out different amounts of light when at the same intensity setting. Sutcliffe (1971) has suggested that this problem can be overcome by sticking small pieces of ND filters over the brighter bulbs. A much better solution would be for the manufacturers to supply the instrument with matched bulbs and to provide a few extra bulbs with the instrument.

Sutcliffe (1971) mentions that the instrument '. . . has generally been found satisfactory as a screening instrument and many glaucomatous and other pathological field defects have been detected by its routine use'. No specific details about the sensitivity or specificity are available and while Sutcliffe has pointed out that the sensitivity of the eye changes with age, he has not provided any base line data for this instrument that would allow optometrists to incorporate an age factor when selecting the intensity of the stimuli for an examination. Part of the problem with providing this sort of information stems from the instrument's lack of calibration facilities. The intensity scale provided does not correspond to any specific stimulus intensity and is unlikely to be the same from one instrument to another.

This instrument does, however, herald another major step forward in the process of developing the ideal optometric field screener. The provision of more stimuli, an ability to adjust stimulus intensity and the facility for detailed kinetic investigation with the Juler scotometer, make it far more versatile than the Harrington–Flocks instrument.

The Globuck screener, the Roberts G11 screener and the DCB screening scotometer

These three instruments are all very similar to the Fincham–Sutcliffe screener. They all use tungsten filament lamps located behind a tangent screen structure and they all suffer from the same problems as the

Fincham–Sutcliffe screener, i.e. difficulty in maintaining exact intensity matches between stimuli and the lack of calibration facilities for either the background or the stimuli, as recommended by the Interprofessional Standards of Visual Field Testing Committee (International Perimetric Society, 1976). A more detailed description of these instruments can be found in Bedwell (1967).

The Visual Field Analyser

The Visual Field Analyser (VFA), or Friedmann Analyser (*see Figure 4.21*), is one of the latest multiple-stimulus static field screeners to be marketed. It is considerably more advanced and sophisticated than its predecessors, the Harrington–Flocks screener and the Fincham–Sutcliffe screener.

Background
illuminator

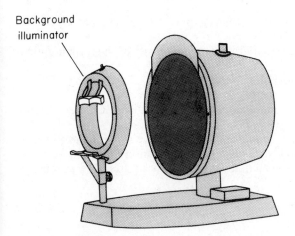

Figure 4.21. The Friedmann Visual Field Analyser Mark I (Clement Clarke)

The stimulus patterns (15 in all) are composed of either two, three or four stimuli and are selected by the rotation of a fenestrated plate situated behind a second, stationary fenestrated plate. Light will only pass through these plates when the fenestrations coincide. A single xenon discharge tube placed within an integrating bowl, the front of which is occluded by the two fenestrated plates, is the light source for all the stimuli. A single flash of this tube results in stimuli being seen at the positions where the fenestrations coincide. The fenestrations are not of equal dimensions, but increase in size towards the periphery to account for the normal gradient in sensitivity across the retina. The larger the hole, the more intense a stimulus will be.

The intensity of all the stimuli can be altered by placing ND filters in front of the xenon bulb. This enables any field defect to be quantitatively measured and also allows the perimetrist to adjust the stimulus intensity for patients of different ages. It is well known that the sensitivity of an average 20 year old is considerably higher than that of an average 80 year old. Clement Clarke provide a table with the Analyser that specifies the neutral density setting that should be used for each age group of patients. It is the only piece of field equipment that provides this essential information. Other manufacturers leave it up to the perimetrists to work out their own set of baseline data.

Although the instrument has an integral background illuminator, it is not provided with a means of either measuring or adjusting the background intensity. While the choice of a black background has made the instrument's findings relatively insensitive to small changes in background illumination, the absence of a light meter that measures the background intensity is a serious omission in what is, generally, a very good piece of equipment.

Greve (1973), in his book on single and multiple static perimetry, gives an extensive list of the advantages and disadvantages of the VFA. Some of his main criticisms are:

1. Too few stimuli, especially in the regions where glaucomatous defects occur (*see Figure 4.22*);
2. No built-in method for standardizing the intensity of the flash illumination;
3. Incorrect choice of hole size in the front plate.

The first criticism is to some extent no longer valid as Clement Clarke have already produced a new VFA which has 98 holes.

The second criticism is based upon some of Greve's own measurements on the amount of light that emanates from the xenon flash in a series of three VFAs. His results showed that the light output differed by as much as

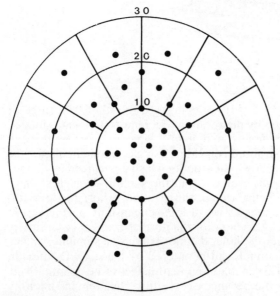

Figure 4.22. The stimulus positions of the Friedmann Visual Field Analyser Mark I

0.2 log units. Greve (1973) proposed that this problem could be overcome by having some built-in means of testing the xenon flash intensity. This, however, is not as easy as it sounds. Since the flash occurs for a period of only 0.5 ms, to monitor its intensity is very difficult. Greve (1973) had to use a high-speed photocell and a storage oscilloscope, hardly items that one is likely to find in the normal optometric practice.

Greve (1973) also measured the degree of fluctuation of intensity with repeated stimulation of the same VFA. He found that as long as the interval between successive stimulations was in excess of 3 s the light output fluctuated by less than ±5 per cent, which, as he points out, is negligible as far as clinical visual field examination goes.

The final criticism was that the sizes of the holes in the front plates are incorrect to compensate for the normal sensitivity gradient of the retina. He claims that the pericentral stimuli are too big and that the stimuli at 15 degrees are too small.

In addition to the increased number of stimuli, the Mark II VFA (*see Figure 4.23*) has a fibre optic system that relays to a chart holder the position of the stimuli being tested. The light that emanates from the ends

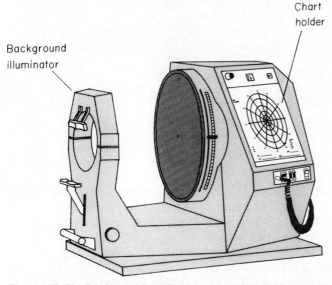

Chart
holder

Background
illuminator

Figure 4.23. The Friedmann Visual Field Analyser Mark II (Clement Clarke)

of the fibre optics can be seen through the field chart and thus any missed points can quickly be marked on the chart. On the Mark I Analyser, the perimetrist has to consult one chart to find out exactly where the stimuli were for each position of the fenestrated plate and then mark the final results down on a second field chart.

The ability of the VFA (Mark I) to detect early glaucomatous defects has been assessed by Greve (1973), who concluded that the instrument failed to detect 17 out of 302 cases with early defects (6 per cent). These failures were largely the result of too few stimuli, a problem which, as mentioned earlier, has been overcome with the development of the Mark II Analyser. The number of false positives in this study was 7 per cent. This instrument has therefore been shown to be both highly sensitive and specific in detecting early glaucomatous damage and is undoubtedly one of the best multiple-stimulus visual field screeners currently marketed.

Computerized equipment

Introduction

Over the last few years the trend in field equipment has been away from mechanically controlled equipment towards electronic control. In its most advanced form, the electronic control is managed by a built-in computer. In addition to relieving the tedium of visual field measurement, computerized perimeters have several other major advantages over conventional equipment:

1. The examination strategy is exactly defined and reproducible. The creators of computer algorithms state their rules explicitly. This results in field defects being reproducible from one examination to another, within the range of variability imposed by the patient, even when the perimetrist changes;
2. They can be operated by technical assistants;
3. The computer system allows flexibility in the testing routine via modification of the programme. For example, should a clinician require to increase the number of points tested or change the location of the points, then the programme can be modified accordingly. With other types of automated field-testing equipment, such as the Friedmann Visual Field Analyser, this can only be achieved by redesigning the instrument;
4. Each instrument can contain a fairly large number of different field examination routines, any one of which can be selected by the clinician. This will enable optimization of any given routine to the suspect pathology, e.g. a separate testing routine can be offered for glaucoma defects and hemianopic defects. The test stimulus for the glaucoma routine would concentrate on the arcuate and nasal areas while the hemianopic routine would concentrate its test stimuli around the midline. Non computerized instruments invariably offer only one routine, which is a type of 'catch-all' programme designed to detect central defects, hemianopic defects and glaucoma defects. By not being specific, they increase the probability, with any given number of stimuli, of failing to detect an early defect;
5. An excess of computer capacity* can be used for novel types of graphical output and to monitor variables such as screen intensity and eye position.

* Many of the current generation of microprocessors are considerably more powerful than required for the relatively simple operation of a perimeter.

Computerized perimeters do have limitations:

1. They do not currently have the ability to take into account data from previous field examinations. This is a particularly important function in hospitals where ophthalmologists are frequently concerned with monitoring any change in field defect that may have occurred since the patient's last visit. Their current technique of using the previous field chart as a template would be extremely difficult to duplicate with a computerized instrument;
2. They require the patient to respond, usually with some form of key press, to each presentation of the target, a task difficult for some patients to perform. This is particularly true for the elderly, who unfortunately constitute that group of the population in whom field defects most often occur. This problem can be overcome if the operator verbally ascertains whether the patient has seen the stimulus and then enters the correct response into the perimeter.

The currently manufactured computerized perimeters fall into two main categories – screening instruments, often designed for use in optometric practices, and research instruments. Instruments that fall into the first category are cheaper and have less flexibility with regard to the stimulus parameters.

The Ocuplot   No longer available.

The Ocuplot is a bowl perimeter with an internal illuminator which controls the light adaptation level of the patient (*see Figure 4.24*). It utilizes an array of small light-emitting diodes (LEDs) as stimuli. While LEDs have a number of advantages, such as speed of response and reliability, they also have some disadvantages, namely their intensity range (limited to about 3–4 log units) and their colour (fixed; green in this instrument). For a screening instrument, these problems are relatively insignificant.

The Ocuplot uses the static mode of examination, presenting one stimulus at a time and then waiting for a response from the patient. There are 127 targets within its programme, the majority of which fall within the central 20 degrees (*see Figure 4.25*). It operates a single programme and displays the results, as the test continues, on a separate LED display attached to the side of the instrument. For each stimulus missed by the patient a side panel LED comes on in a corresponding position to the missed bowl stimulus. By placing a chart over this display, it is possible to map out any scotoma with a pen. Any missed points are automatically retested.

During the examination, the patient views a red fixation target that incorporates an automatic fixation monitor. If the patient looks away from this target during the examination then its colour changes to green and a small light on the control panel comes on to inform the operator that fixation is lost. This type of system has the advantage over other fixation monitors of giving immediate feedback to the patients about their fixation accuracy. The perimetrist can alter the sensitivity of the fixation monitor

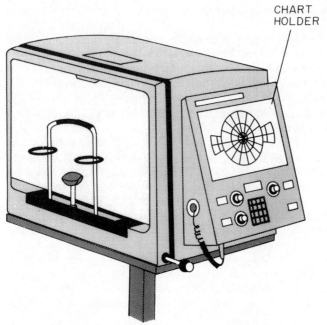

CHART
HOLDER

Figure 4.24. The Ocuplot perimeter (Coherent Radiation)

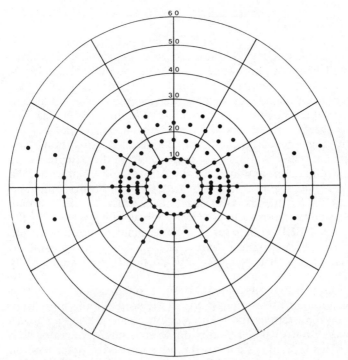

Figure 4.25. The stimulus positions of the CFA 120, an early version
of the Ocuplot

and can set the instrument such that either the programme is interrupted when fixation is lost or the programme continues irrespective of fixation accuracy.

The designers of the Ocuplot have matched many of the parameters of the stimuli and background to those of the Goldmann perimeter. The LEDs have been masked down to 1 mm^2 (Goldmann size II target) and can be presented at any of the four Goldmann intensity levels (10, 31.8, 100 and 318 cd/m^2). The background intensity, which is continuously variable, is set by the manufacturers to equal that of the Goldmann (10 cd/m^2) when at its zero position. There is, however, no light meter provided with the Ocuplot and thus the perimetrist is unable to check these settings or make adjustments to the background intensity when the instrument is used in a room with some ambient illumination.

The problem, experienced with all visual field equipment that utilize a large number of discrete light sources, of matching the intensities of the individual stimuli has been overcome by matching the LEDs prior to assembly. Coherent Radiation provide a number of spare LEDs with the instrument should one need replacing. As the average life expectancy of an LED is 10 years of continuous use, it is doubtful that these spares will be needed.

The Ocuplot takes no account of the gradient of sensitivity that occurs across the retina. This means that if the peripheral targets (55 degrees from the fovea) are set at the average threshold (*see* Greve, 1973) the central targets (5 degrees from the fovea) will be approximately 2 log units above threshold. A patient would therefore need a very severe central field loss before he would fail to detect the central stimuli. Decreasing the intensity of the targets to make the instrument more sensitive in the central field would result in patients failing to detect many of the peripheral targets.

An early version of the Ocuplot, the CFA 120, has been evaluated by Johnson and Keltner (1980)*. They compared the results of the CFA 120 with those of a Goldmann perimeter with which both kinetic and static measures of the visual field were taken. The results from 99 eyes, of which 54 had a defect, showed the CFA 120 to have a 90.7 per cent detection rate and a 17.9 per cent false alarm rate. Thus, while the CFA 120 may be considered as having a fairly good detection rate, its false alarm rate is exceedingly high and would result in many unnecessary referrals. To put these figures in perspective, the Friedmann Mark I Field Analyser has a 94 per cent detection rate and a 7 per cent false alarm rate.

Automatic Tangent Screen

The Automatic Tangent Screen is a single-stimulus static device that attaches to the wall of the consulting room. Behind and shining through its front screen are 114 LEDs arranged in the pattern shown in *Figure 4.26*. Depending upon the programme selected, 90, 64 or 32 of these LEDs are individually presented to the patient who responds to each seen presentation by depressing a small hand-held button. Each missed point is

---

* The CFA 120 differs from the Ocuplot in that the stimulus and background intensities are not as accurately calibrated and the LEDs are not matched prior to assembly.

automatically retested at the end of the selected programme. After the test has finished, the results are displayed on a matrix of LEDs in the upper left hand corner of the screen. By placing a field chart over this matrix, it is possible to plot the location of the missed points.

The instrument does not have any background illumination system, but can monitor the screen illumination with the aid of a small photocell situated behind the front panel. It is possible, therefore, by having some control over the room illumination to adjust the background intensity to some predetermined level. Unfortunately, the photocell has not been calibrated and thus, while it allows the perimetrist to arrive at the same intensity level for each examination, it does not indicate exactly what that intensity level is.

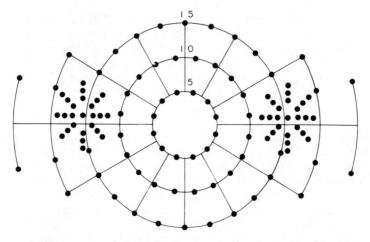

Figure 4.26. The stimulus positions of the Automatic Tangent Screen (Computation)

The stimulus duration and interstimulus interval can be set to any value from 0.1 to 9.9 s, but are preset at the beginning of the examination to 1.0 and 0.5 s, respectively. Any person who wishes to use values different to the preset ones would have to change these everytime the instrument was used. The stimulus intensity level can also be adjusted from its preset value. During this procedure one of the LEDs comes on to give the perimetrist an idea of how bright the stimulus is at each of the settings. All the LEDs are matched prior to assembly so that their intensities are equivalent when driven by the same current. The instrument is provided with a wand that enables the perimetrist to kinetically measure the extent of any scotoma.

While this instrument has certain novel features not seen in other tangent screens, such as its recording system, it has two major disadvantages. First, the luminance of the screen and the stimuli are not specified as recommended by the Interprofessional Standards Committee (International Perimetric Society, 1976). Second, the instrument does not take into account the gradient of sensitivity that occurs across the retina, which means that in normal operation it will either be insensitive to defects close to the macula or give a large number of missed points in the periphery (*see* the section on Ocuplot).

The Fieldmaster

The Fieldmaster is a bowl perimeter (*see Figure 4.27*) with a built-in light meter that allows the perimetrist to set both the background and stimulus intensities. The background intensity is normally set at 31.5 asb with the aid of the meter, but can be set to other values that range from 0 to considerably above 31.5 asb. The use of a light meter that displays its results in apostilbs is a considerable improvement over many other instruments because it not only allows the perimetrist to use other than the standard background illumination, but also to specify that illumination.

The stimulus intensity is normally set at 400–450 asb, but can be set to values from 0 to greater than 1000 asb. This flexibility allows the

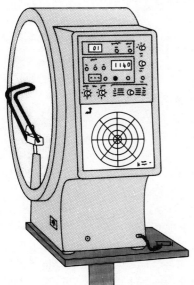

Figure 4.27. The Fieldmaster perimeter (Synemed Inc.)

perimetrist to measure the depth of any scotoma and to make adjustments for the normal change in sensitivity that occurs with age. The manufacturers do not, however, provide any normative data with this perimeter that would allow the operator to simply dial in the correct values. It is left up to the perimetrist to establish the normative data.

The Fieldmaster utilizes a fibre optic system to convey the light from a central lamp to the individual test points within the globe (*see Figure 4.28*). This type of arrangement results in all the stimuli being presented at the same intensity and makes it impossible, within any single programme, to take into account the normal gradient of sensitivity across the retina. The instrument, therefore, suffers from the same problem as the Ocuplot in that it either has to be set so as to be insensitive to central defects or set so that subjects fail to detect many of the peripheral targets. A solution to this problem, recommended by the distributors, is that the central field is tested at one intensity and the peripheral field at another. While this is possible with the expensive version of this instrument, which has a total of 10 programmes, one of which tests the central field and another the peripheral field, it is not possible with the cheaper version. In any case, the solution can only be considered as a compromise since the gradient of sensitivity is a continuously varying function.

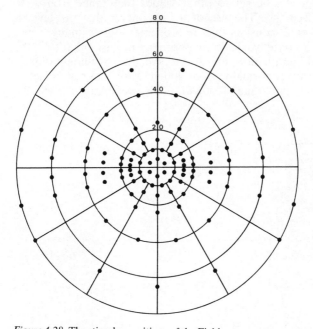

Figure 4.28. The stimulus positions of the Fieldmaster

The stimulus presentation time and the interstimulus interval can be set by the operator within the range of 0.3–4.3 s. The Fieldmaster does not, however, keep to these values throughout the test period, but randomly varies them in order to stop the patient from automatically responding as a result of a temporally repetitive stimulus. The values set by the operator are the average values for the test duration. While the variation in presentation time should have no effect upon the measured sensitivity, as even the shorter presentations are in excess of the retinal summation time, there does not seem to be any advantage in varying both the stimulus duration and the interstimulus interval. In fact, Greve (1973) recommends that stimulus presentation times be kept as short as possible so as to reduce any effects that might be produced as a result of eye movements.

The instrument contains an eye fixation monitor, composed of four light sensors situated around the fixation point. These sensors are masked down such that they view only the region around the eye being examined. If the patient moves or changes fixation during the examination to such an extent that the output of one of these sensors alters beyond some established

Don't know what's happening until test over - Px may not have understood.

range, then the instrument bleeps and discontinues the examination until the patient refixates or repositions. The sensitivity of this device can be varied by the perimetrist via a knob on the control panel which adjusts the range over which the photocells can alter without triggering the warning system. The UK distributors state that at the zero setting of the knob (range −3 to +3) a bleep would occur for an eye movement in excess of 2 degrees. The nature of the fixation monitor means that it is not only sensitive to eye position, but also to head position. If the patient should move his head while maintaining accurate fixation, then the monitor will interrupt the programme. Once interrupted, it may be found impossible to reposition the patient with sufficient accuracy to enable the test to continue without recalibrating the fixation monitor (this requires a simple button press). Fortunately, this recalibration does not initiate the whole programme; the test continues from where it was interrupted.

The results of the examination are plotted automatically on heat-sensitive paper. Unfortunately, the plotter marks each point on the chart as it is seen. Thus, at the end of the examination the perimetrist has to ~~Disadv~~ carefully examine the chart to check that none of the points have been missed. It would have been much simpler if the instrument had adopted the more conventional approach of charting missed points rather than seen ones.

As mentioned previously, the Fieldmaster comes in two forms, of which the more expensive contains a series of 10 programmes that allow the perimetrist to specifically examine the peripheral or central fields, to screen for glaucoma, etc. The cheaper instrument offers a single catch-all type programme. Both instruments automatically recheck missed points and allow the perimetrist to individually retest any point or to recheck again the missed points at a higher intensity.

The Fieldmaster has been evaluated by Johnson and Keltner (1980). They used the expensive version of the instrument and tested the peripheral field at one intensity setting and the central field at a lower one (635 asb peripheral and 200 asb central). They compared their results with those obtained with the Goldmann perimeter with which a combined kinetic and static procedure was adopted. Their findings on 1019 eyes of which 436 had a defect, showed the Fieldmaster to have a 96.1 per cent detection rate and a 4.7 per cent false alarm rate. These figures demonstrate that when the Fieldmaster is used in this way it is a very reliable instrument.

The Octopus

The Octopus was one of the earliest computerized perimeters made commercially available and has thus been a pioneer in the field. It is a bowl instrument that controls the background intensity and the stimulus intensity. Stimuli are projected onto the inside surface of the bowl as in the Goldmann instrument. The use of of a projected stimulus allows a particularly large range of stimulus parameters, it being possible to have a target of almost any size, any colour, at any intensity.

Its technique of recording is entirely different to that of the previously discussed instruments in that it establishes the threshold at each point in the visual field rather than testing at some pre-determined supra threshold level. In order to achieve this, it presents each stimulus 4–7 times in what is known as a repetitive bracketing strategy. Briefly, this means that if the target was seen on the first presentation its intensity is reduced for the second one and vice versa. The intensity for the third presentation is based upon the first and second responses, etc. The intensity steps are reduced as the number of presentations at each stimulus position increases. Although each stimulus is presented a number of times, each of these presentations is randomly mixed with the presentations of other stimuli. It is thus impossible to predict the position of the next stimulus. The repetitive bracketing technique obviously deals with individual variability and the gradient of sensitivity in any patient. The disadvantage is that it takes a long time to perform an examination.

∴ accounts for retinal sensitivity

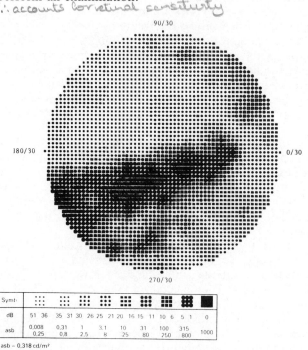

Figure 4.29. One of the types of field plot obtainable with the Octupus perimeter (Interzeag)

The number of points tested is dependent upon the programme selected. Specific programmes are available for glaucoma screening, general screening, precision perimetry of a 12 × 12 degree area, etc. The instrument tests the reliability of a patient by retesting certain points and comparing values. Fixation of the patient is monitored by a close circuit television that relays to the operator's console an image of the patient's eye. Its print-out device is an electronic typewriter with a special type face which is capable of producing the type of plot given in *Figure 4.29*. Finally, the perimeter has the ability to store a patient's results on a mass storage device such that, at a subsequent visit, they can be recalled for comparison.

The Perimetron (Coherent Radiation)

The Perimetron is currently one of the most sophisticated of all the perimeters. It contains no less than three microprocessors and can do almost anything possible with a standard bowl perimeter, only automatically. Stimuli are projected onto the inside surface of the bowl as in the Goldmann and Tubinger instruments (*see* the previous comments on the Octopus).

The Perimetron is currently the only computerized perimeter that has the facility to use <u>kinetic and static</u> techniques of field examination. The programming of the kinetic technique is so sophisticated that the instrument has the capability of completely plotting any scotoma automatically, i.e. once a scotoma has been found, the instrument will gradually work its way around it, plotting, in the case of an isolated scotoma in the peripheral field, both from the periphery to the central region of the field and from the centre to the periphery.

The perimeter <u>monitors eye fixation automatically</u> as well as providing a telescope device for the operator to view the patient during the examination. The automatic monitor, which is accurate to ±3 degrees on its 'fine' setting, is an eye movement recorder which is set up by the operator prior to the beginning of the field examination. If problems arise with a subject on the 'fine' setting, it is recommended that the 'coarse' one be used, which has an accuracy of ±10 degrees. The value of such a monitor is exceedingly limited. While this criticism has been levelled at the Perimetron, it is equally valid for all the other perimeters that offer automatic fixation monitors. In fact, it is to the credit of Coherent Radiation that they admit to the deficiency of this system and provide the operator with the <u>alternative of direct viewing</u>.

The instrument plots its data out automatically on an XY plotter for analysis by the perimetrist.

References

ARMALY, M. F. (1971). Visual field defects in early open angle glaucoma. *Transactions of the American Ophthalmological Society*, **69**, 147

AULHORN, E. and HARMS, H. (1967). Early visual field defects in glaucoma. In *Glaucoma Symposium*, p. 15. Edited by W. Leydhecker. S. Karger, Basle

AULHORN, E. and HARMS, H. (1972). Visual Perimetry. In *Handbook of Sensory Physiology*, Vol. 7/4, p. 102. Edited by L. M. Hurvich and D. Jameson. Springer-Verlag, New York

AULHORN, E. and KARMEYER, H. (1976). Frequency distribution in early glaucomatous visual field defects. In *Documentum Ophthalmologica Proceedings Series, Second International Visual Field Symposium, Tubingen*, Vol. 14, p. 75. Edited by E. Greve. Dr W. Junk, The Hague

BEDWELL, C. H. (1967). Instrumentation for visual field investigation. *Ophthalmic Optician*, **7**, 328, 382, 447, 520, 566, 616

DRANCE, S. M., WHEELER, C. and PATULLO, M. (1967). The use of static perimetry in the early detection of glaucoma. *Canadian Journal of Ophthalmology*, **2**, 249

GREVE, E. L. (1973). *Single and Multiple Stimulus Static Perimetry in Glaucoma; The Two Phases of Perimetry*. Dr W. Junk, The Hague

GREVE, E. L. and VERDUIN, W. M. (1976). Detection of early glaucomatous damage. Part 1. Visual field examination. In *Documentum Ophthalmologica Proceedings Series, Second International Visual Field Symposium, Tubingen*, Vol. 14, p. 103. Edited by E. Greve. Dr W. Junk, The Hague

HAGEDOORN, A. and VAN DEN BOSCH, Ch. (1955). A double projection campimeter. *American Journal of Ophthalmology*, **40**, 891

HARRINGTON, D. O. (1956). *The Visual Fields*. Henry Kimpton, London

HARRINGTON, D. O. and FLOCKS, M. (1959). The multiple-pattern method of visual field examination. A five year evaluation of its effectiveness as a visual screening technique. *Archives of Ophthalmology*, **61**, 755

HENSON, D. B. (1980). Visual field equipment. A critical review, part I. *Optician*, **180**, Oct 31st, 14

INTERNATIONAL PERIMETRIC SOCIETY (1976). First interprofessional standard for visual field testing, 1975. *Journal of the American Optometric Association*, **47**, 829

JOHNSON, C. A. and KELTNER, J. L. (1980). Comparative evaluation of the Autofield–I, CFA–120 and Fieldmaster Model 101–PR automated perimeters. *Ophthalmology*, **87**, 777

REED, H. and DRANCE, S. M. (1972). *The Essentials of Perimetry, Static and Kinetic*. Oxford University Press, London

ROCK, W. J., DRANCE, S. M. and MORGAN, R. W. (1973). Visual field screening in glaucoma. *Archives of Ophthalmology*, **89**, 287

SCHOESSLER, J. P. and UNIACKE, C. A. (1977). Standardisation of the Bausch and Lomb Autoplot tangent screen. *American Journal of Optometry and Physiological Optics*, **54**, 782

SLOAN, L. (1961). Area and luminance of test objects as variables in examination of the visual field by projection perimetry. *Vision Research*, **1**, 121

SUTCLIFFE, R. L. (1971). Techniques of visual field examination and the design of new instrumentation. *Ophthalmic Optician*, **11**, 308, 315, 361, 409

TATE, G. and LYNN, J. (1977). *Principles of Quantitative Perimetry*. Grune and Stratton, New York

5
Keratometers

Principles and theory of keratometry

Keratometers (also known as ophthalmometers) are instruments used to measure the radius of curvature of the anterior corneal surface. This measurement is utilized to fit contact lenses and to monitor corneal changes produced through the wear of contact lenses. Keratometers are also occasionally used to assist in the recognition of certain corneal abnormalities and to check the radii of curvature of both hard and soft contact lenses.

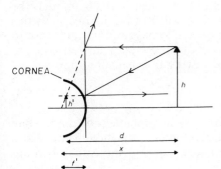

Figure 5.1. The optical principles of the keratometer

Keratometers utilize the reflective properties of the cornea in order to measure its radius of curvature. By measuring the size of an image, formed by reflection from the cornea, of an object of known size and position, a measurement of the radius can be calculated. The theory of keratometry is depicted in *Figure 5.1*, where it can be seen that the magnification of the image is equal to h'/h where h' equals the size of the image and h the size of the object. By similar triangles, it can be seen that

$$\frac{h'}{h} = \frac{f'}{x} = \frac{-r}{2x} \tag{5.1}$$

Transposing equation (5.1), we find that the radius of the cornea is

$$r = 2mx \qquad (5.2)$$

where m equals the magnification of the image.

The magnification of the corneal image is of the order of 0.03 for a keratometer mire (test object) positioned approximately 15 cm from the eye. This magnification, or rather minification, makes the mire image so small that a compound microscope has to be used in order to accurately measure its size (*see Figure 5.2*). Because the object of known size (or mire) of the keratometer is invariably attached to the objective of this

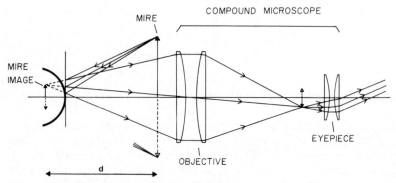

Figure 5.2. An optical diagram of the compound microscope of a keratometer

compound microscope, its image will only be seen in focus through the microscope when the mire is a given distance, d, from its image. If this distance is large, then the position of the mire image will be very close to the focal point of the corneal mirror, i.e. d will be approximately equal to x, in which case equation (5.2) can be rewritten as equation (5.3).

$$r = 2md \qquad (5.3)$$

Equation (5.3) is known as the *approximate* keratometer equation, while equation (5.2) is known as the *exact* keratometer equation. Since d is a constant for any particular instrument, the radius of the cornea is proportional to the magnification.

In theory, the size of the mire image could be measured by simply placing a measuring graticule within the microscope. However, a problem arises in keratometry due to the continual movement of the patient's eye. Everytime the eye moves, the mire image moves, which makes it exceedingly difficult to measure with any degree of accuracy.

This problem has been successfully overcome by the use of a doubling system. The principles of one type of doubling system, the biprism, are depicted in *Figure 5.3*. Here it can be seen that the amount of doubling produced by a biprism is dependent upon the position of the prism with respect to the objective lens. If this distance is reduced, the extent of doubling increases and if it is increased, the extent of doubling decreases.

By varying the position of the biprism, the amount of doubling can be made to equal the size of the image. By then recording the position of the prism, the exact size of the image can be calculated. This technique overcomes the problem of eye movements because the two images stay in alignment when the eye moves. The appearance of a mire, such as that

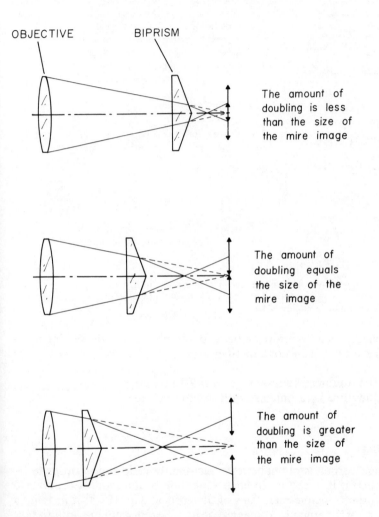

OBJECTIVE   BIPRISM

The amount of doubling is less than the size of the mire image

The amount of doubling equals the size of the mire image

The amount of doubling is greater than the size of the mire image

Figure 5.3. The amount of doubling produced by a biprism, placed between the objective of a keratometer and the mire image, is dependent upon the position of the biprism

shown in *Figure 5.4*(a), when viewed through a keratometer with varying degrees of doubling, is given in *Figures 5.4*(b), (c) and (d). Keratometers that incorporate the principle just described are known as variable doubling keratometers. Alignment can also be obtained by altering the size of the mires, while the amount of doubling is kept constant.

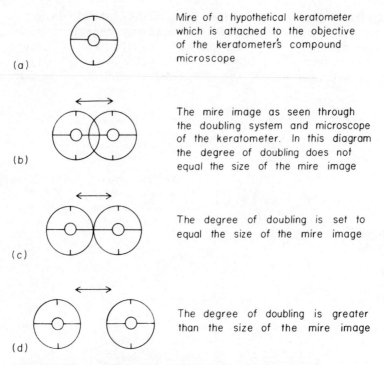

(a)   Mire of a hypothetical keratometer which is attached to the objective of the keratometer's compound microscope

(b)   The mire image as seen through the doubling system and microscope of the keratometer. In this diagram the degree of doubling does not equal the size of the mire image

(c)   The degree of doubling is set to equal the size of the mire image

(d)   The degree of doubling is greater than the size of the mire image

Figure 5.4. The appearance of a hypothetical mire when seen through a keratometer with varying degrees of doubling. The arrows indicate the axes of the keratometer and the doubling system

Keratometers can therefore be divided into two groups depending upon the technique they use to obtain alignment:

1.   Variable doubling keratometers with fixed mires;
2.   Variable mire keratometers with fixed doubling.

Astigmatism

The average cornea is not spherical, but slightly toric and in order to be fully specified it is necessary to have a measure of the radius of curvature along both the principle meridians of the cornea. The effect of imaging a mire with a toric cornea is to magnify it by different amounts in different meridians, the maximum and minimum magnifications being along the two principle meridians of the cornea. The object mire shown in *Figure 5.4*(a) will appear as in *Figure 5.5*(a) after it has been reflected by a toric cornea the principal meridians of which lie at 45 and 135 degrees. While the two elliptical images can be brought into aposition with each other by varying the amount of doubling or size of the mire (*see Figure 5.5*(b)), correct alignment can only be obtained by rotating the keratometer until its doubling axis coincides with one of the cornea's principal meridians. By then varying the doubling or size of the mires, it is possible to align the

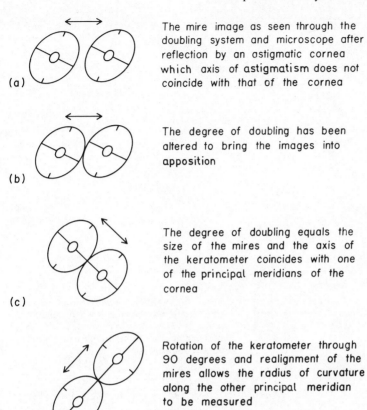

(a) The mire image as seen through the doubling system and microscope after reflection by an astigmatic cornea which axis of astigmatism does not coincide with that of the cornea

(b) The degree of doubling has been altered to bring the images into apposition

(c) The degree of doubling equals the size of the mires and the axis of the keratometer coincides with one of the principal meridians of the cornea

(d) Rotation of the keratometer through 90 degrees and realignment of the mires allows the radius of curvature along the other principal meridian to be measured

Figure 5.5. The appearance of the mires after reflection from an astigmatic cornea

mire images as shown in *Figures 5.5*(c) and (d). With these two measurements the toric cornea can be fully specified in a manner such as that shown below:

7.4 mm along 135 degrees
7.8 mm along 45 degrees

One and two position keratometers

Because the axes of a toric surface are always at 90 degrees to each other, some instrument manufacturers have designed keratometers that incorporate two separate doubling systems which operate in mutually perpendicular meridians. Although these instruments still have to be rotated about their anterior and posterior axes in order to find one of the principal meridians of a toric cornea, once this position has been found no further rotation of the instrument is necessary in order to obtain a radius measurement along the second principal meridian. This type of keratometer is known as a one position instrument, while keratometers that

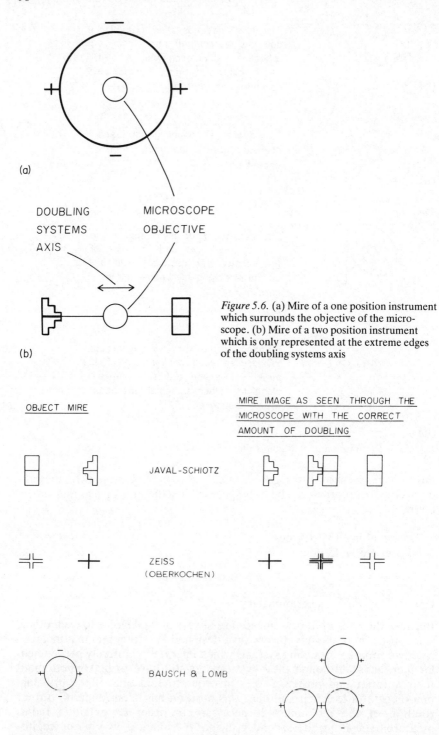

(a)

DOUBLING   MICROSCOPE
SYSTEMS   OBJECTIVE
AXIS

(b)

Figure 5.6. (a) Mire of a one position instrument which surrounds the objective of the microscope. (b) Mire of a two position instrument which is only represented at the extreme edges of the doubling systems axis

OBJECT MIRE

MIRE IMAGE AS SEEN THROUGH THE MICROSCOPE WITH THE CORRECT AMOUNT OF DOUBLING

JAVAL-SCHIOTZ

ZEISS
(OBERKOCHEN)

BAUSCH & LOMB

Figure 5.7. Three types of commonly found mires

require rotation through 90 degrees in order to measure the second principal meridian are known as two position instruments.

While the principal meridians of a toric lens are always at 90 degrees to each other, those of the cornea need not be. This is because the corneal surface more closely approximates a toric ellipse than a toric surface and when an off-axis measurement is taken of a toric ellipse the principal meridians need not necessarily be at 90 degrees to each other.

Until now we have considered the keratometer mire as a single, large object which surrounds the optical axis of the keratometer. While many one position keratometers have such mires, the majority of two position instruments only represent the mire at the extreme edges of the doubling system's axis (*see Figure 5.6*). The reason for this is that it is only these extreme edges that are used to obtain alignment. The design of the object mire varies considerably from instrument to instrument. *Figure 5.7* gives the patterns of three commonly found designs.

Area of cornea used during keratometry

It can be seen from *Figure 5.8* that the light reflected from the cornea comes not from its centre, but from two small areas on either side of the instrument axis. The size of these areas is dependent upon the effective aperture of the keratometer's objective. The principles upon which keratometry is based assume that a spherical surface exists between these

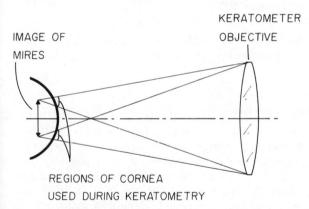

Figure 5.8. The two regions of the cornea from which the mires are reflected into the keratometer

two areas. This need not be the case. It is, in fact, well known that the normal cornea is not spherical, but flattens off towards its periphery. Because of this and because different keratometers reflect their mires from different regions of the cornea, two readings of the same cornea with two different keratometers may not give the same radius. Lehmann (1967) has calculated the exact separation of the corneal regions, used with different keratometers, for a whole series of different corneal radii. Some of his results are shown in *Figure 5.9*.

That keratometers only record from two small areas of the cornea must make the optometrist wary of relying on *K* readngs as the sole indicator of corneal distortion during aftercare visits. It is theoretically feasible to have a small area of corneal irregularity that lies between the two areas measured with the keratometer. In this situation, the keratometry readings

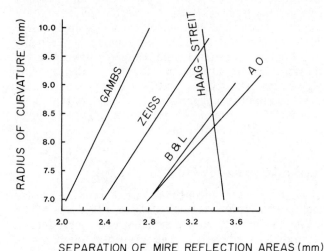

SEPARATION OF MIRE REFLECTION AREAS (mm)

Figure 5.9. The separation of the corneal areas used with different keratometers. After Lehmann (1967)

would be normal while the cornea itself was distorted. Similarly, it is possible to have corneal irregularities beyond the area of cornea measured with a keratometer.

The dioptric scales on keratometers

In addition to giving a measurement of the cornea's anterior radius of curvature, all currently produced keratometers also give an estimate of the total corneal power – i.e. the combined power of the front and back surfaces. To do this, keratometer manufacturers have had to assume certain values for the cornea's back surface. The majority of them have accepted the values adopted by Listing and Helmholtz who, in the production of a schematic eye, stated that the total corneal power could be reduced to a single curved surface with a refractive index equal to 1.3375 (Emsley, 1963). It should be recalled that the true refractive index of the cornea is 1.376. Subsequent work by Gullstrand has shown that a more accurate estimate of corneal power is obtained if a refractive index of 1.333 is used rather than 1.3375.

The main value of these dioptric scales is to allow the contact lens practitioner to calculate the amount of residual astigmatism, this being defined as the amount of astigmatism that exists after a patient has been fitted with a hard spherical contact lens. Because the refractive index of the tears is very close to that used by the keratometers to calculate total corneal power, the amount of astigmatism measured with the keratometer will be very close to that neutralized by the liquid lens when a spherical contact lens is fitted. Thus, by comparing the amount of astigmatism measured with the keratometer with the ocular refraction, the practitioner can rapidly assess the value of any residual astigmatism.

Currently, the majority of keratometers still use a refractive index of 1.3375 in order to give an estimate of total corneal power, although some now use 1.336 or even 1.332. While these different values give different estimates of the total corneal power, they do not result in any significant differences in the calculated amounts of corneal astigmatism (Stone and Francis, 1980). Since keratometers use different refractive indices, it is less confusing to specify a cornea using millimetres of radius rather than dioptres.

The calibration of keratometers

When the theory of keratometers was described earlier two equations were derived; the exact keratometer equation (5.2) and the approximate keratometer equation (5.3). Both of these equations are based on paraxial theory. Bennett (1966) has questioned whether the utilization of paraxial theory is valid in keratometry where the radii of the surfaces being measured are so very small. He takes a hypothetical instrument, which approximates a Bausch and Lomb keratometer, and calculates the angle, for a whole series of both convex and concave radii, subtended by the mire image at the entrance pupil of the keratometer's microscope using:

1. The approximate keratometer equation;
2. The exact keratometer equation;
3. A ray tracing technique.

He finds that while all three conditions give an approximately linear relationship between corneal radius and angle subtended at the microscope objective, the use of paraxial theory results in an error of about 4–5 per cent. This means that a cornea of true radius 8.0 mm would be recorded as having a radius of curvature of 7.7 mm. The manufacturers of keratometers overcome this problem by calibrating their instruments on a series of known radii similar to those of the cornea. By doing this they reduce the errors induced by the use of paraxial theory to an insignificant level for any particular form of surface. If, however, a keratometer calibrated on convex surfaces is used to measure the radius of curvature of a concave surface, a large error will be introduced. While this is obviously not a problem when it comes to measuring the radius of curvature of the cornea, it is a problem when the keratometer is used to check the radii of curvature of contact lenses (*see* pp. 104–106).

Eyepiece focusing errors in keratometry

In order for the majority of keratometers to give an accurate reading of the corneal curvature, it is essential that the eyepiece of the instrument be correctly focused. To facilitate this a graticule is invariably placed within the instrument upon which the eyepiece should be focused prior to making a radius measurement. The types of errors induced by incorrect focusing of the eyepiece can be reduced or eliminated by careful design of the keratometer's optics. The Gambs keratometer, Zeiss (Oberkochen) ophthalmometer and the Rodenstock C-BES keratometer have all been designed to eliminate eyepiece focusing errors. Before going on to describe how this has been achieved, it would be advantageous for the reader to understand in more detail the exact nature of eyepiece focusing errors.

Let us consider what happens when the eyepiece of the instrument is positioned too far out. In this situation, the whole instrument has to be repositioned closer to the patient's cornea in order for the operator to see the mires already in focus. This repositioning of the instrument results in two distinct errors. The first is due to the mires being positioned closer to the patient. When this occurs (*see Figure 5.10*), the size of the mire image

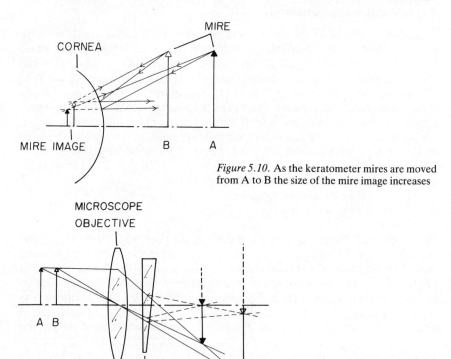

Figure 5.10. As the keratometer mires are moved from A to B the size of the mire image increases

Figure 5.11. The amount of doubling alters as the mire image moves from A to B

formed by the corneal mirror increases and, in order to overcome this error, the mires have to be moved closer towards the axis of the instrument or the degree of doubling has to be decreased.

The second error is produced because the degree of doubling in an instrument which uses a prism placed on the eyepiece side of the objective, such as the Bausch and Lomb keratometer or the Javal–Schiotz keratometer, alters with the distance from the mire image to the objective lens. This is demonstrated in *Figure 5.11*, where it can be seen that, as the mire image is brought closer to the objective lens, i.e. from point A to B, the magnification of the mire image increases and the original coincidence setting of the keratometer is upset. To overcome this error, the mires would again have to be positioned closer to the optical axis of the instrument or the degree of doubling would have to be reduced. The product of the two errors is therefore larger than either of the errors in isolation.

The magnitude of the error induced by incorrect eyepiece focusing can be exceedingly large. Rabbetts (1977) has measured it on a series of commonly encountered keratometers. Some of his results are shown in *Table 5.1*. It should be recalled, while inspecting this table, that hard contact lenses are manufactured to a radius tolerance of 0.02 mm and fitted in 0.05 mm steps.

TABLE 5.1. The magnitude of the focusing errors produced in some commonly found keratometers. (After Rabbetts, 1977)

Instrument	Radius of test ball (mm)	Errors produced in measured radius (mm) Lens generating error					
		+10.00	+7.00	+5.00	−5.00	−7.00	−10.00
		Artificial myopia			Artificial hyperopia		
American Optical	6.5			−0.06	+0.065		
CLC	8.0			−0.05	+0.11		
	9.0			−0.11	+0.07		
Baush and	6.5			−0.06	+0.05		
Lomb	8.0			−0.07	+0.06		
	9.0			−0.20	+0.14		
Topcon OM-2	6.5	−0.03	−0.03		0.00		+0.01
	8.0	−0.07	−0.04		+0.05		+0.08
	9.0	−0.10		−0.07	+0.06		+0.10
Guilbert–Routit	6.5	−0.07		−0.04	+0.05		+0.10
(Javal–Schiotz)	8.0	−0.08		−0.04	+0.08		+0.14
	9.0	−0.13		−0.03	+0.07		+0.12
Haag–Streit	6.5		−0.14			+0.12	
(Javal–Schiotz)	8.0		−0.19	+0.13	+0.08	+0.20	
	9.0		−0.19			+0.21	
Gambs		no measurable difference					

The first error, the one due to the mires being positioned too close to the cornea, can be eliminated by optically imaging the mires at infinity (collimated mires). This is shown in *Figure 5.12*, where each mire is placed at the focal point of a convex lens. It can be seen from this figure that as the mires are moved from A to B the size of the image produced by the corneal mirror remains unaltered.

The second error can be eliminated by one of two techniques. The first of these uses two parallel glass plates in front of the objective as a variable doubling device, rather than a movable prism behind the objective. This technique was first mentioned by Helmholtz in the nineteenth century, but is not, to my knowledge, incorporated in any currently manufactured keratometers. A diagram of the arrangement of the glass plates is given in

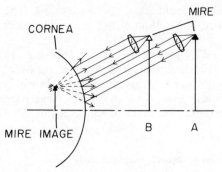

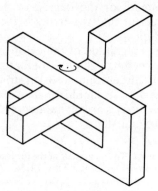

Figure 5.12. Ray diagram showing how, when the mires are placed behind positive lenses that image them at infinity, the mire image does not alter when the mire is moved from A to B

Figure 5.13. Helmholtz doubling system

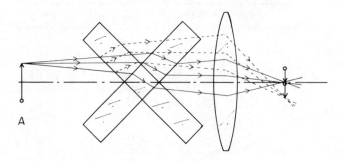

HELMHOLTZ   MICROSCOPE
DOUBING SYSTEM   OBJECTIVE

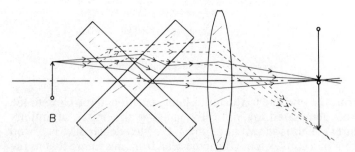

Figure 5.14. With the Helmholtz type of doubling system the alignment of the mires is not upset when the mire image moves from A to B

Figure 5.13 and a second diagram of the principles of this type of keratometer is given in *Figure 5.14*.

The second technique for eliminating this error, which is used in both the Gambs and the Zeiss (Oberkochen) keratometers, utilizes the telecentric principle, which can be explained most easily by referring back to *Figure 5.11*. This figure shows that as an object is moved from position A to

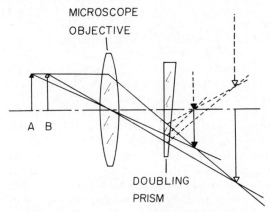

Figure 5.15. When the doubling prism is placed beyond the focal point of the objective the alignment of the mires is upset with the movement of the mire image from A to B

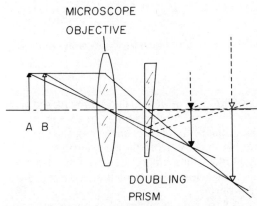

Figure 5.16. When the doubling prism is placed at the focal point of the objective the alignment of the mires is not upset by the movement of the mire image from A to B

position B, its image becomes larger and the initial coincidence setting is upset so that either the mires have to be moved closer to the axis of the keratometer or the degree of doubling has to be reduced. If the prism is placed beyond the focal point of the objective lens, as shown in *Figure 5.15*, then as the target is moved from A to B, the image again becomes larger and the coincidence setting is disturbed. However, coincidence is regained in this situation by moving the mires away from the axis or by increasing the degree of doubling, i.e. the exact reverse to that previously necessary. If the prism is placed at the focal point of the objective lens, as shown in *Figure 5.16*, then the coincidence setting is unaltered by the movement of the object from A to B.

To eliminate focusing errors with the telecentric principle, as outlined above, it is essential that the doubling prism does not move along the axis of the keratometer, i.e. the instrument has to have either variable mires or a doubling system different to that previously outlined. The type of doubling system used in these keratometers will be discussed later, when the individual instruments are described in more detail.

The Rodenstock C-BES keratometer has neither collimated mires nor a telecentric viewing system and yet its focusing error is zero. This has been achieved by making the error due to positioning the mires too close to the eye cancel out the error due to the microscope being placed too close to the eye. This type of instrument is known as a compensated keratometer. Removal of the error by compensation can be achieved by at least two different techniques. The first is to place positive lenses in front of the mires such that images of the mires are produced at a point behind the patient's head. The second is to place a positively powered lens in front of a Helmholtz-type doubling system such that the corneal image of the mires, as seen by the objective lens, lies behind the patient's head. The positioning of these intermediary images is important and has to be carefully calculated for the focusing error to be totally eliminated. The C-BES keratometer uses the latter of the two systems.

Use of the keratometer to measure the radii of curvature of contact lenses

Hard lenses

The back central optic radius of hard contact lenses can be measured with the aid of a small attachment to the keratometer similar to that shown in *Figure 5.17*. To reduce the reflections from the front surface of the lens to a point where they do not interfere with those from the back surface, a drop of water is placed between the contact lens holder and the lens. Because the refractive index of water is fairly close to that of the lens, very little light will be reflected from this interface.

Since keratometers are calibrated for convex surfaces, a conversion scale will have to be used when measuring back optic radii (*see* pp. 98–99). Many of the instrument manufacturers provide these scales with the keratometer. If, however, one is not available, the practitioner can produce one with the aid of a few hard contact lenses of known back central optic radius. He or she should measure the back central optic radius of each contact lens with the keratometer and draw a graph of keratometer reading versus the known radius of the contact lens. This graph, which should be a straight line, can then be used to convert subsequent keratometer readings by simply looking up the contact lens radius that corresponds to the keratometer reading.

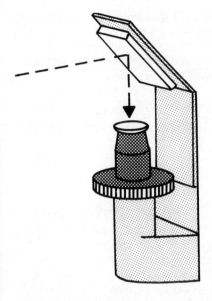

Figure 5.17. Keratometer attachment for the measurement of contact lens radii

It is possible to get an attachment for the Rodenstock keratometer that enables the practitioner to measure both central and peripheral contact lens radii. The mirror of this attachment can be set at angles other than 45 degrees so as to direct the keratometer axis towards the periphery of the lens.

Soft lenses

The keratometer can also be used to check the radii of curvature of soft contact lenses. It is preferable, when taking this measurement, to have the lens immersed in a small cell which contains saline solution (*see Figure 11.19*), as this will prevent the lens from drying out and consequently altering its radius during the measurement process. It is important to recalibrate the keratometer when measuring soft lens radii in this way since the use of the saline will result in a difference between the keratometer scale and the true contact lens radius. This calibration can be performed with a series of hard contact lenses of known back central optic radii. Each lens should be placed, one after the other, in the saline solution for measurement with the keratometer. By plotting known hard contact lens radius versus keratometer scale reading, a graph can be drawn that will allow subsequent readings from soft lenses to be converted.

Loran (1980) has pointed out that many keratometers do not have a sufficiently large measuring range to be able to measure the steeper soft lens radii. A solution to this problem is to place a low-power positive lens (+1.25 D; Hartstein, 1973) in front of the microscope objective. With this lens in place, it will be necessary to recalibrate the keratometer in the manner just outlined. The amount of light reflected from an interface is dependent upon the refractive indices of the two boundary media. The closer they are to each other, the smaller will be the percentage of reflected light. Unfortunately, the refractive index of saline is fairly close to that of

soft contact lenses and the mire images will therefore be very faint. A
further problem with this technique is that both surfaces of the contact lens
produce mire images of approximately the same intensity and it can, with
plus lenses in the range of +0.25 to +6.00 D, be almost impossible to
differentiate between the two reflections (Chaston, 1978).

Types of optical systems incorporated in keratometers

Most of the currently produced keratometers fall into one of the following
three categories:

1. Fixed doubling, variable mires;
2. Variable doubling, fixed mires;
3. Telecentric.

In the following pages, three instruments are described, one from each
category mentioned above. A list of the keratometers which have similar,
if not identical, optical designs is included in each description. This section
ends with a brief description of the Humphrey Auto Keratometer, which is
capable of measuring the corneal radius without the optometrist having to
align a set of mires. However, this instrument is still based upon the same
principles as the other keratometers, i.e. it measures the size of the mire
image.

Javal–Schiotz type keratometers*

The Javal–Schiotz (*see Figure 5.18*) keratometer is a fixed doubling,
variable mire, two position instrument. The mires are attached to the front

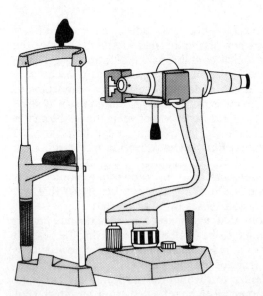

Figure 5.18. A Javal–Schiotz keratometer (Guilbert Routit)

* Javal–Schiotz keratometers are made by Guilbert Routit, Haag–Streit, Inami, Jewel and
Sbisa.

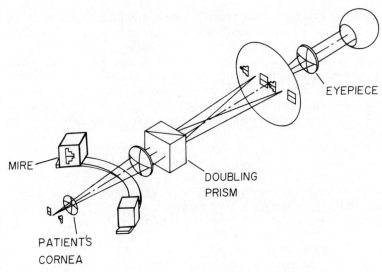

Figure 5.19. Javal–Schiotz keratometer. After Mohrman (1981)

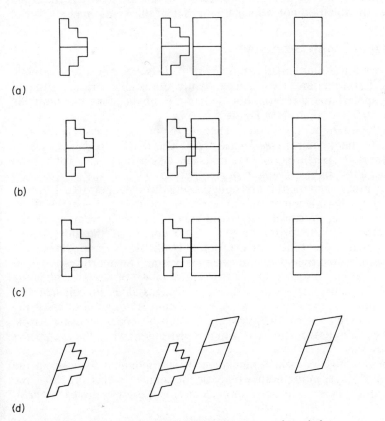

(a)

(b)

(c)

(d)

Figure 5.20. Appearance of the Javal–Schiotz mires as seen through the microscope for the conditions described in the text

of small light boxes which, via a gearing arrangement, are made to move equally in opposite directions along a circular arc, the centre of curvature of which corresponds to the patient's eye. Doubling is achieved with a Wollaston prism placed behind the objective lens (*see Figure 5.19*). The whole instrument can rotate about its optical axis to enable measurement along any meridian. Provided care is taken in setting up the instrument and in ensuring that the eyepiece is correctly focused, this keratometer is capable of providing results comparable, in accuracy, to that of other keratometers.

The original mire pattern of the Javal–Schiotz keratometer is shown in *Figure 5.7*. The stepped mire has a green filter over it while the square one is covered by a red filter. These filters help the practitioner to recognize when the mires overlap as any area of superimposition appears yellow. The appearance of the mire images as seen through the doubling system of the microscope is shown in *Figure 5.20* for the conditions where:

(a)   The mire separation is too large;
(b)   The mire separation is too small;
(c)   The mire separation is correct;
(d)   The mires are viewed after reflection by an astigmatic cornea, the axes of which do not coincide with that of the keratometer.

Bausch and Lomb keratometer*

The Bausch and Lomb instrument (*Figure 5.21*) is a one position, variable doubling keratometer. Two independently adjustable prisms, situated behind a special aperture stop, double the mire image along two mutually perpendicular meridians (*see Figure 5.22*).

When the instrument is correctly aligned, the operator sees three images of the instrument's mires (*see Figure 5.23*). The first is produced by light passing through aperture C and the vertically displacing prism. The second is produced by light passing though aperture D and the horizontally displacing prism, and the third by light passing through apertures A and B. Back and forth movement of the vertically doubling prism results in movement of the vertically displaced image, while movement of the horizontally doubling prism results in movement of the horizontally displaced image. The central image formed by the light passing through A and B is unaffected by movement of either prism. The apertures A and B act like a Schiener disc and double the central image of the mire when the intermediate image, produced by the objective lens, does not coincide with the focal point of the eyepiece lens. This system is designed to assist the operator in judging when the microscope is out of focus. Focusing errors, as previously discussed, still exist with this instrument when the eyepiece is incorrectly set.

In cases of high corneal astigmatism, it is impossible to position the central mire single along both astigmatic meridians. In this situation, the instrument needs to be focused for each meridian prior to a measurement

* Optically similar instruments are made by American Optical, Bolor, Inami, Kelvin, Topcon and Sbisa.

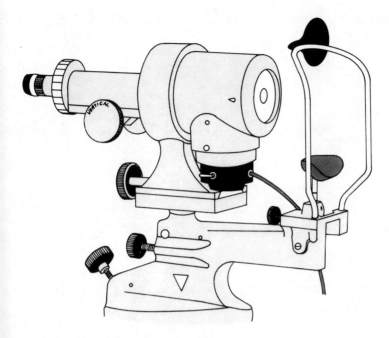

Figure 5.21. The Bausch and Lomb keratometer

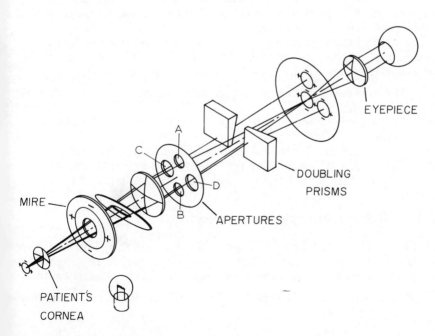

Figure 5.22. Optics of the Bausch and Lomb keratometer. After Mohrman (1981)

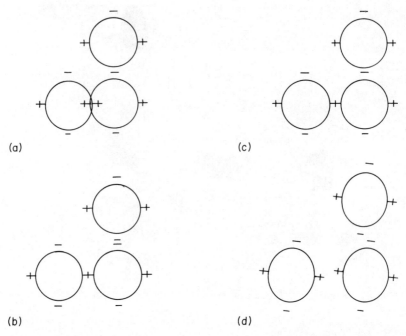

(a)   (c)

(b)   (d)

Figure 5.23. Appearance of the Bausch and Lomb keratometer mires as seen through the microscope for the conditions described in the text below

in that meridian. One position instruments assume that the two astigmatic axes are at 90 degrees to each other. Because of the geometry of the cornea, this is not always the case (*see* pp. 95–97).

The mire of the Bausch and Lomb keratometer is shown in *Figure 5.7*. The images of the mire as seen through the doubling systems of the keratometer are shown in *Figure 5.23* for the conditions where:

(a)   The vertical doubling is correct and the horizontal doubling is insufficient;

(b)   The vertical doubling is too great and the horizontal doubling is correct;

(c)   The vertical and horizontal degrees of doubling are correct;

(d)   The mires are viewed after reflection by an astigmatic cornea, the axes of which do not coincide with that of the keratometer.

Zeiss (Oberkochen) ophthalmometer*

The Zeiss ophthalmometer (*Figure 5.24*) is a variable doubling, two position keratometer. The optics of the instrument have been designed so as to eliminate errors due to poor focusing. This has been achieved by:

1.   Placing the mires behind positive lenses which image them at infinity (collimated mires);

---

* An optically similar instrument is made by Gambs.

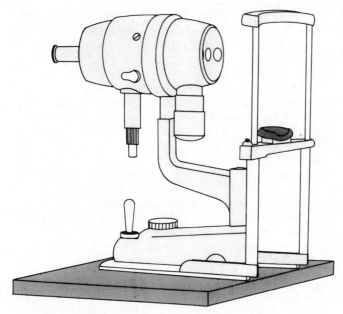

Figure 5.24. The Zeiss (Oberkochen) keratometer

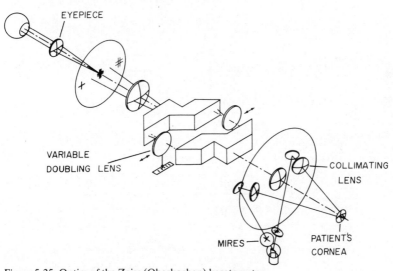

Figure 5.25. Optics of the Zeiss (Oberkochen) keratometer

2. Placing the doubling system at the focal point of the objective lens
    (telecentric principle).

The previously described variable doubling system, that of a prism
moving along the axis of the instrument, is incompatible with the telecentric principle, which requires that the doubling system remains at the focal
point of the objective lens. Zeiss have therefore developed a new type of
doubling system which is composed of two lenses that move in opposition

to each other and move perpendicularly to the optical axis of the instrument (*see Figure 5.25*). The amount of doubling produced by these lenses, i.e. their prismatic effect, is proportional to the amount they are displaced from the optical axis.

The Zeiss ophthalmometer has a rather unusual recording system. The instrument has two scales; one records the radius of curvature and dioptral power of the front surface of the cornea, while the other reads the amount of front surface astigmatism. In use, the astigmatism scale should first be zeroed and a reading along one of the principle meridians made by rotating the knob that alters the radius of curvature scale. The instrument should then be rotated through 90 degrees and the mires brought back into alignment by turning a second knob that alters the astigmatism scale. The operator can then read off from the two scales a prescription for the cornea, in dioptres. For UK optometrists who have been taught to take keratometer readings in millimetres of radius, it is essential that the astigmatic scale remains at zero for both readings.

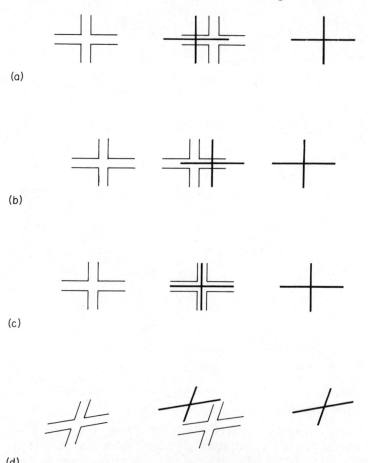

(a)

(b)

(c)

(d)

Figure 5.26. Appearance of the Zeiss (Oberkochen) keratometer mire as seen through the microscope for the conditions described in the text on p. 113

Optically, the instrument is a joy to use. The collimated mires have a much brighter image than those of many other instruments, which makes alignment easier. The freedom from focusing errors means that movements of the patient are less troublesome, for although they may result in a blurring of the images, they do not affect alignment. This freedom from focusing errors is valuable when it comes to assessing the fit of soft contact lenses. With this instrument, the optometrist can view the reflections from the front surface of a lens while it is on the eye and can see if the lens lifts from the cornea (steepens its radius) after a blink. While this measurement can also be made with keratometers that have focusing errors, it is occasionally difficult to decide whether a change in the alignment of the mires is the result of a radius change or a change in the distance between the keratometer and the eye.

The mires of the Zeiss ophthalmometer are shown in *Figure 5.7*. The appearances of the mire images through the doubling system of the microscope are shown in *Figure 5.26* for the conditions where:

(a)   The amount of doubling is too large;
(b)   The amount of doubling is too small;
(c)   The amount of doubling is correct;
(d)   The mires are viewed after reflection by an astigmatic cornea, the axes of which do not coincide with that of the keratometer.

The Humphrey Auto Keratometer

The Humphrey Auto Keratometer measures the corneal radius of curvature at three locations along the horizontal meridian. The central measurements are taken with the patient looking straight into the instrument, while the peripheral ones are made with the patient looking 13.5 degrees nasally and 13.5 degrees temporally. With the aid of an in-built computer, the Auto Keratometer converts the peripheral readings into a measurement of the corneal shape factor (the degree to which it flattens off in the periphery) and an estimate of the vault height. It also calculates the position of the corneal apex and gives a conformance factor. The conformance factor tells the optometrist how well the measured cornea matches a theoretical cornea, the parameters of which are stored in the instrument. If the measured cornea conforms very badly with the theoretical one then this indicates an irregularly shaped cornea.

The Humphrey Auto Keratometer does not require the optometrist to align any mire images. Once correctly positioned, the keratometer measures the cornea automatically. The mire of the Humphrey instrument is composed of three infra-red emitting diodes arranged in a triangular shape. In place of the observer it uses a solid state detector that records the exact position of each diode image after reflection from the cornea. The in-built computer uses this information to calculate the size of the mire image and the radius of curvature of the cornea. The speed with which these detectors operate is so fast that eye movements do not create a problem for the measurement system. The instrument does not, therefore, contain a doubling system.

Currently, Humphrey instruments are developing the computer programme, contained within the instrument, to provide further information that may be of value to the contact lens practitioner. Whether this additional information will be of sufficient value to offset the cost of the Humphrey instrument is yet to be seen. There is no doubt, however, that this instrument is a very good example of how electronics can overcome some of the optical problems encountered in the design of optometric instruments.

Other techniques of corneal measurement

It has often been said that if sufficient information were available about the topography of a patient's cornea, then it should be possible to select a contact lens that would have an ideal fitting relationship without going through the normal fitting procedures. The keratometer in its basic form only gives information about the central radius of curvature. It does not tell the optometrist anything about the way in which the cornea flattens towards its periphery or the exact location of the corneal apex (point of shortest radius).

In an attempt to overcome this problem, several keratometers are marketed with an optional attachment that allows the optometrist to measure the curvature of the cornea off the visual axis. The attachment to the Bausch and Lomb keratometer (Topogometer) consists of an illuminated fixation light that can be moved along two axes, both of which are perpendicular to the axis of the keratometer. Scales are attached to the Topogometer which indicate, in mm, the amount of decentration of the visual axis from the optical axis of the keratometer at the corneal surface. The Topogometer can aid the optometrist in the fitting of contact lenses by giving an estimation of the degree of peripheral flattening and the position of the corneal apex.

Information about the topography of the cornea can also be obtained with a photokeratoscope. This instrument finds its origins back in the nineteenth century with a much simpler device known as Placido's disc. This disc is essentially a flat, black, round plate upon which are attached a series of concentric white rings (*see Figure 5.27*). In the centre of the plate is a peephole in which is placed a positive lens. Images of the concentric rings (mires) are viewed by the optometrist after reflection from the cornea through the positive lens. Any irregularities in the cornea display themselves as irregularities in the mire images. In its basic form, Placido's disc is only sensitive to gross irregularities of the corneal surface, such as may occur in certain pathologies. As a contact lens fitting aid, therefore, it would have no use. However, Gullstrand modified Placido's disc by attaching a camera to it that was capable of photographing the mire images. His instrument was called a photokeratoscope. By carefully measuring the size and shape of the mire images, Gullstrand was able to calculate the topography of the cornea. The theory behind the photokeratoscope is exactly the same as that for a keratometer.

Ludlam and Wittenberg (1966) describe many of the shortcomings of Gullstrand's photokeratoscope. One of these is curvature of the image plane. With a large aperture system, such as that found in the photokerato-scope, the image becomes curved and it becomes impossible to obtain all the rings in focus at the film plane. This problem can be overcome by curving the object, i.e. by placing the rings on the inside of a bowl rather than on a flat plate.

A second problem is alignment of the patient's cornea with the photo-keratoscope. Most measurements of corneal curvature are taken along the line of sight which is assumed to coincide with the corneal apex. It has already been shown by Mandell and St. Helen (1971), however, that the corneal apex does not necessarily coincide with the line of sight or any other common reference point.

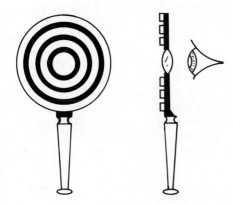

Figure 5.27. Placido's disc

The third and final problem that Ludlam and Wittenberg (1966) mentioned relates to the analysis of the data. They found that the quality of the image produced was such that accurate measurement was not always possible.

Wesley–Jessen Inc. have produced a photokeratoscope, known as the PEK, that resolves many of the problems outlined by Ludlam and Wittenberg (1966) (*see Figure 5.28*). The mires of this instrument are placed on the inside of an elliptical bowl so that, for the average cornea, a flat image will be produced in the film plane.

In addition to this, Townsley (1967, 1970) has developed a new mathematical treatment of the photokeratogram that does not require it to be taken symetrically about the apex of the cornea. Measurements from the photokeratogram are entered into a computer which calculates the parameters of the conic section that best fits the cornea along both its flattest meridian and one at 90 degrees to it. Wesley–Jessen use this data, along with information about the refractive error and the type of fitting relationship wanted by the practitioner, to calculate the parameters of a contact lens. The PEK instrument, with allied computer data reduction systems, undoubtedly provides a precision of corneal measurement currently unobtainable with any other piece of commercially available equipment. However, contact lens fitting requires more than a precise knowledge of corneal contour because even with this instrument it is impossible to guarantee a successful fit.

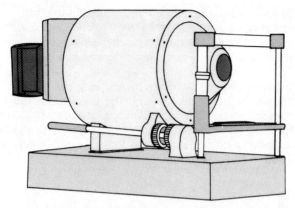

Figure 5.28. The PEK photokeratoscope (Wesley–Jessen)

The final technique that has been used successfully to obtain information about corneal topography is called stereophotography. This technique, which was developed within the field of cartography, allows the mapping of complex shapes such as the cornea from two photographs taken simultaneously. It requires the cornea to be made opaque, which can only be achieved by anaesthetizing it and coating it with a fine powder. Understandably, this rather unpleasant procedure makes the technique unacceptable for contact lens practice.

Referrences

BENNETT, A. G. (1966). The calibration of keratometers. *Optician*, **151**, 317

CHASTON, J. (1978). The verification of the optical dimensions of the soft lens. In *Soft Contact Lenses: Clinical and Applied Technology*, p. 457. Edited by M. Ruben. Balliere Tindall, London

EMSLEY, H. H. (1963). *Visual Optics*, Vol. 1, 5th Edn. Hatton Press, London

HARTSTEIN, J. (1973). *Questions and Answers on Contact Lens Practice*. Mosby, St Louis

LEHMANN, S. P. (1967). Corneal areas used in keratometry. *Optician*, **154**, 261

LORAN, D. F. C. (1980). The verification of soft contact lenses. In *Contact Lenses*, Vol. II, p. 469. Edited by J. Stone and A. J. Phillips. Butterworths, London

LUDLAM, W. M. and WITTENBERG, S. (1966). The effect of measuring corneal toroidicity with reference to the line of sight. *British Journal of Physiological Optics*, **23**, 178

MANDELL, R. B. and St. HELEN, R. (1971). Mathematical model of the corneal contour. *British Journal of Physiological Optics*, **26**, 183

MOHRMAN, R. (1981). The keratometer. In *Clinical Ophthalmology*, Vol. 1, Ch. 60, p. 1. Edited by T. D. Duane. Harper and Row, Hagerstown

RABBETTS, R. B. (1977). Comparative focusing errors of keratometers. *Optician*, **173**, April 28th, 28

STONE, J. and FRANCIS, J. (1980). Practical optics of contact lenses and aspects of contact lens design. In *Contact Lenses*, Vol. 1, p. 91. Edited by J. Stone and A. J. Phillips. Butterworths, London

TOWNSLEY, M. G. (1967). New equipment and methods for determining the contour of the human cornea. *Contacto*, **11(12)**, 72

TOWNSLEY, M. G. (1970). New knowledge of the corneal contour. *Contacto*, **14(3)**, 38

6
Slit lamps

Introduction

Slit lamps are used in the examination of the anterior segment of the eye and adnexa. They are particularly valuable in contact lens work where they allow the practitioner to perform a careful examination of the cornea, conjunctiva and lids both before contact lens fitting and as part of the aftercare routine. Slit lamps consist of a relatively low-power binocular microscope, through which the clinician views the patient's eye, and a light source that illuminates the patient's eye (*see Figure 6.1*). In most modern instruments, the microscope and light source are coupled so that the light shines on the same part of the eye that the microscope is focused. This coupling greatly facilitates examination of the eye.

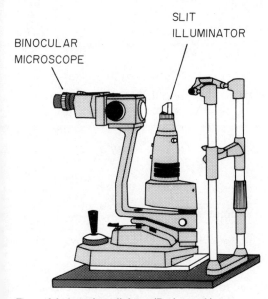

Figure 6.1. A modern slit lamp (Rodenstock)

The instrument is called a slit lamp because, in its normal mode of operation, the light source produces a thin vertical slit of light at the eye. When this slit of light shines along a different axis to that of the microscope, the clinician sees a section of the living eye (*see Figure 6.2*). Normally transparent tissues, such as the cornea and lens, can be seen when they fall in the path of the slit of light because the cells and fibres

Slit of light passing
through the cornea
and lens

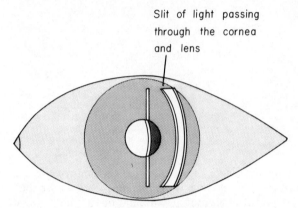

Figure 6.2. Section of the eye as seen with a slit lamp

within these tissues scatter a small amount of the incident light. The effect is similar to that seen at the cinema when cigarette smoke passes through the projector's beam. By moving the instrument around and altering the angle between the lamp and the microscope, the clinician is able to examine most of the anterior segment of the eye.

In the first half of this chapter, the following aspects of the basic slit lamp are described:

1. Slit lamp microscopes;
2. Illumination systems;
3. Mechanical coupling.

The second half of the chapter deals with 'special slit lamp techniques and attachments' and includes:

1. Pachometry;
2. Fundus examination;
3. Gonioscopy;
4. Tonometry;
5. Laser photocoagulation;
6. Measuring visual acuity in patients with hazy media.

Slit lamp microscopes

Slit lamp microscopes are designed to have long working distances, i.e. the distance between the microscope objectives and the eye. This not only gives some working room should the clinician wish to hold open the patient's lids or remove a foreign body from the eye, but also leaves room for certain accessories to be attached to the slit lamp such as tonometers and pachometers (*see* later section of this chapter). The magnification of slit lamp microscopes is usually within the range of ×6 to ×40. At higher magnifications, the small and often uncontrollable movements of the patient's eye make the image jump around so much that an examination cannot be performed satisfactorily. This range of magnifications and the large working distance mean that compound rather than simple microscopes have to be used. In their most basic form, compound microscopes are composed of two optical elements, an objective and an eyepiece. A diagram of the optical arrangement of these two elements is given in *Figure 6.3*(a). While they are shown in this figure as two simple positive lenses, in reality the eyepiece and occasionally the objective are composed of a series of lenses in order to reduce aberrations.

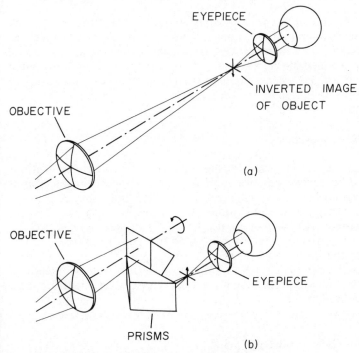

Figure 6.3. (a) Optical arrangement of the objective and eyepiece in a compound microscope. (b) In the slit lamp microscope a pair of prisms is used to reinvert the image

One of the problems of compound microscopes is that the final image is inverted with respect to the object. To overcome this, slit lamp microscopes use a pair of prisms (*see Figure 6.3*(b)) between the objective and the eyepiece to reinvert the image. The eyepieces and prisms can usually be rotated around the optical axis of the microscope such that the instrument can be adjusted for practitioners with different interpupillary distances. This arrangement, which is the same as that found in a prism binocular, also has the advantage of shortening the length of the microscope.

Most slit lamps provide a range of magnifications. The lower magnifications are used to locate any abnormalities, while the higher ones allow a more detailed examination of any abnormality. This range of magnification is produced via either one or a combination of the following four techniques:

1. The use of different objectives;
2. The use of different eyepieces;
3. The Littmann–Galilean telescope principle;
4. With a zoom system.

The use of different objectives

This is one of the oldest and possibly still the most frequently used technique for obtaining different magnifications. The different objectives are usually placed on a turret type of arrangement that allows them to be fairly rapidly changed during an examination. The system is usually limited to two sets of objective lenses due to the confinements of space in and around the objective area of the slit lamp.

The use of different eyepieces

This technique is usually used to augment the range of magnifications provided by other techniques, although on some of the cheaper slit lamps it is the only means of changing the magnification. It is not a very convenient technique as it requires the practitioner to pull out the current eyepieces and replace them with ones normally kept in a drawer attached to the instrument table. It is unusual for more than two pairs of eyepieces to be provided with the slit lamp and hence this technique alone provides a very limited range of magnifications. In combination with two sets of objectives, it can provide four different magnifications, which is sufficient for most types of examination.

The Littmann–Galilean telescope principle

The Galilean magnification changer, as developed by Littmann (1950), is a completely separate optical system that sits neatly between the objective and eyepiece lenses and does not require either of them to change. It provides a larger range of magnifications than the previously mentioned techniques, typically five, via a turret arrangement which is completely enclosed within the microscope's body. It is called a Galilean system because it utilizes Galilean telescopes to alter the magnification. Galilean telescopes have two optical components, a positive and a negative lens arranged in the manner shown in *Figure 6.4*. Parallel light both enters and leaves the system and undergoes some degree of magnification which is dependent upon the power and separation of the two lenses. The Galilean telescope fits within the standard slit lamp microscope along with a relay lens in the manner shown in *Figure 6.5*.

By reversing the order of the lenses in the telescope, a different magnification can be achieved (this time a minification) without altering

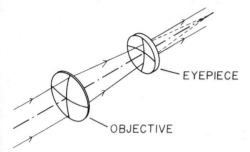

Figure 6.4. Galilean telescope

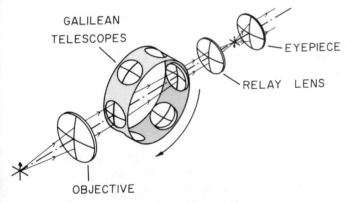

Figure 6.5. Galilean telescope magnification changer

any other optical elements. Thus, with the provision of two Galilean telescopes, both of which are reversible, four different microscope magnifications are available. Typically, slit lamps using this system also allow both telescopes to be removed from the optical path of the microscope, thereby increasing the range of magnifications to five.

Zoom systems

Recently, two of the more expensive slit lamps (Nikon and Zeiss (Oberkochen)) have been produced with zoom systems that allow a continuously variable degree of magnification. The Nikon instrument contains the zoom system within the objective of the microscope and offers a range of magnifications from ×7 to ×35.

Illumination systems

The objective of the slit lamp illumination system is to produce a bright, evenly illuminated, finely focused, adjustable slit of light at the eye. To this end, virtually all slit lamp manufacturers have adopted the Koeller illumination system. It is optically identical to that of a 35 mm slide projector with the exception that a variable aperture slit takes the place of the slide and the projector lens has a much shorter focal length. Reflectors are occasionally positioned behind the lamp in order to increase the amount of light that passes through the condensers. The radius of curvature of any reflector is made to coincide with the filament of the bulb so as to re-image the filament back on itself. This arrangement ensures that there are no additional unwanted images of the filament.

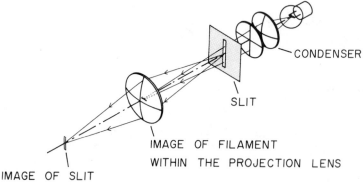

Figure 6.6. The Koeller illumination system

   In the Koeller illumination system, the filament of the bulb is imaged by the condenser lenses at or close to the projector lens (*see Figure 6.6*). The projector lens forms an image of the slit at the eye. The diameter of the projection lens is usually fairly small. This has two advantages: first, it keeps the aberrations of the lens down, which results in a better quality image; second, it increases the depth of focus of the slit and thereby produces a better optical section of the eye. While the optics of the condenser are not as critical as that of the other elements of the slit lamp, care must be taken in their design so as not to introduce too much chromatic aberration, which will tend to cause fringes at the slit image. A reduction of this aberration is normally achieved by using two or more lenses in the condenser system.
   The width of the slit is controlled, usually in a continuous manner, via a mechanical arrangement. Its height is adjusted either in discrete steps with a series of apertures placed in front of the slit or continuously with a screw arrangement (*see Figure 6.7*). Different filters can be inserted into the illumination beam either to reduce the illumination when a wide slit aperture is used or to excite fluorescence in the eye when fluorescein has been used. In addition to this, rotation of the slit away from the vertical meridian is often available and, occasionally, the ability to tilt the

projection system about a horizontal axis is provided. These two additional degrees of freedom are included to assist in the examination of the fundus and the angle of the anterior chamber (*see* later sections). For a review of many of the facilities incorporated in the majority of currently manufactured slit lamps, the reader is referred to Sasieni (1981).

The light source used in virtually all slit lamp illumination systems is a tungsten filament bulb. For safety reasons, they are run on relatively low voltages. Some slit lamps can now be obtained with halogen-filled bulbs which have a considerably larger light output. These bulbs are useful in slit lamp photography and in instances where special techniques, such as

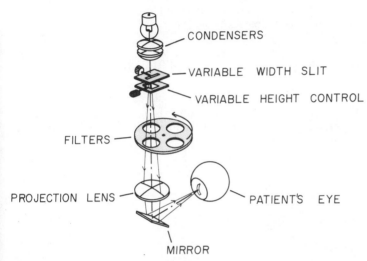

Figure 6.7. Typical slit lamp illumination system

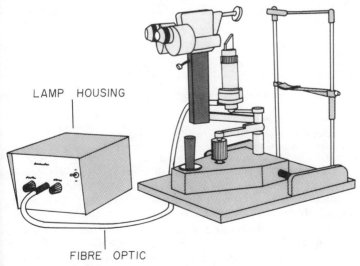

Figure 6.8. The Diag slit lamp (Clements Clarke)

pachometry, are practised. For normal slit-lamp examination more than enough light is available from a standard filament bulb, provided the optics of the projection system are well designed.

The Diag slit lamp (*see Figure 6.8*) has an unusual illumination system in that it uses a fibre optic to convey the light from a high-power halogen bulb, housed in a special fan-cooled box, to the slit lamp. This arrangement has been adopted in order to decrease the weight of the slit lamp and to allow it to be hand held by the practitioner, thereby doing away with the need for an instrument table and chin rest (Bedwell, 1978). Because of problems in keeping the microscope steady when it is hand held, the magnification of this slit lamp is kept low, at ×6. The instrument can be stand mounted in the same manner as other slit lamps and its magnification increased by changing its eyepieces.

Mechanical coupling of microscope and illumination system

The microscope and illumination system of all currently produced slit lamps are linked together around a common axis of rotation that coincides with their focal planes (*see Figure 6.9*). This means that the point where the

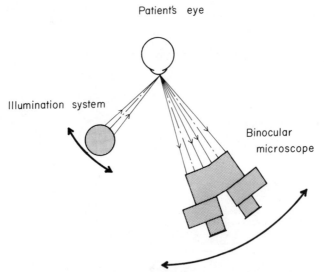

Figure 6.9. Aerial view of a slit lamp which shows how the illumination system and the binocular microscope are focused at the same point. The arrows indicate how the illumination system and the microscope can be rotated around the point at which they are focused

microscope is focused coincides with the point where the illumination system is focused. It allows either the microscope or the illumination system to be rotated around this axis without changing the focus. (The Zeiss (Oberkochen) 10SL is an exception to this rule, the microscope being fixed in the straight ahead position (Davey, 1977).) The coupling of the microscope and illumination systems in this way is advantageous when using the slit lamp for routine examination of the anterior segment of the eye. It is, however, a problem when certain specific forms of examination (scleratic scatter, retro-illumination) or specific techniques of examination (gonioscopy, *see* a later section p. 131) are required. To enable these other techniques to be used, it is usually possible to disassociate the illumination and viewing systems so that the illumination system is focused to one side of the point where the microscope is focused. It is only rarely possible, however, to independently alter the focus of either system.

Movement of the microscope and illuminator towards or away from the eye and from side to side is usually achieved via a joystick arrangement, while up and down movement is obtained via some sort of screw device that moves the whole illumination and viewing systems up and down relative to the chin rest. With these two controls, it is relatively easy to focus on any part of the anterior globe or adnexa.

The illumination system of a slit lamp has to be able to pass relatively easily from one side of the microscope to the other. To allow this, the projection system is normally arranged along a vertical axis, with either a mirror or a prism finally reflecting the light along a horizontal axis (*see Figure 6.7*). The use of a narrow prism or mirror means that when necessary, such as in examination of the fundus, the illumination axis can be made to almost coincide with the viewing axis without obstructing the field of view.

Corneal thickness gauge (pachometer)

The measurement of corneal thickness has recently received a great deal of attention due to its potential ability to monitor corneal integrity in contact lens patients. While there are many different techniques of measuring corneal thickness (Ehlers and Kruse Hansen (1971) mention five, all of which have at sometime been suggested within the literature), the majority of measurements being taken today utilize the technique developed by Juillerat and Koby (1928) of measuring the apparent thickness of the optical section.

The popularity of this technique is largely the result of the commercial availability of a pachometer attachment for the Haag–Streit 900 major slit lamp. There follows a description of this attachment and some of the suggested modifications to it.

Description of the pachometer attachment

The pachometer hangs over the objectives of the microscope from a post attached to the microscope body. The left objective is occluded by the pachometer while the right one has two glass plates with parallel sides placed in front of it (*see Figure 6.10*). These plates rest one on top of the other with the junction between them situated so as to horizontally bisect the objective. The top block can be rotated while the bottom one is fixed and positioned so that its faces are normal to the axis of the microscope. When the top plate is rotated, the image seen through it is displaced by an amount dependent upon the angle of rotation. The resultant view through the microscope is of two corneal optical sections whose relative separation can be adjusted by rotation of the top plate. A measurement of the corneal thickness is made by simply aligning the outer surface of the epithelium of one section with the inner surface of the endothelium of the other. The amount of rotation necessary to achieve this is read off directly from a scale attached to the pachometer, which is calibrated in mm of corneal thickness.

To assist in the accuracy of making this setting, Haag–Streit have developed a special eyepiece that removes from the field of view half of the

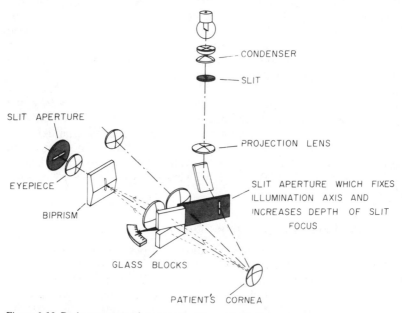

Figure 6.10. Pachometer attachment to the Haag–Streit slit lamp

two optical sections (*see Figure 6.11*). The eyepiece is a conventional ×10 one with the addition of two components – a small horizontal slit placed on the observer's side of the eyepiece, and a biprism, apex horizontal, positioned on the patient's side. The slit is positioned (*see Figure 6.12*) such that it is imaged, by the eyepiece and objective lenses, in the plane of the glass blocks. This arrangement limits the light that passes through the lower half of the biprism and slit to the upper glass block as well as the light that passes through the upper half of the biprism and slit to the lower glass block. The apex of the biprism is imaged by the objective at the cornea. Thus, when correctly focused, only the upper half of the cornea is seen through the lower half of the biprism and only the lower half of the cornea through the upper half of the biprism. The combined effect of the slit and biprism is to allow only the upper half of the cornea to be seen through the top glass block and the lower half of the cornea through the bottom glass block – i.e. half of the two optical sections have been removed from the field of view.

As the apparent thickness of the cornea varies with the angle between the slit lamp and the microscope, it is essential to set this at some predetermined value before a measurement is made. With the Haag–Streit slit lamp this angle should be 40 degrees.

With this pachometer it is difficult to know when the incident beam is normal to the corneal surface. Measurements taken with it at any other angle will result in a thicker-than-true corneal measurement. To overcome this problem, Mishima and Hedbys (1968) introduced a modification to the Haag–Streit pachometer which consists of two small light sources placed a further 40 degrees to the left of the slit. Images of these light sources will be

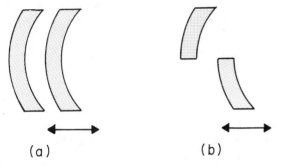

(a)   (b)

Figure 6.11. The appearasnce of the cornea (a) without and (b) with the special eyepiece

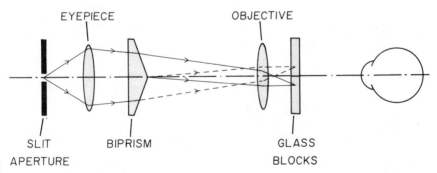

Figure 6.12. The optical arrangements of the glass blocks, biprism and slit aperture in the Haag–Streit pachometer

seen through the microscope after reflection at the cornea and will be coincident with the front surface of the cornea when the slit beam is normal to the corneal surface. When the beam is at any other angle, they will be seen as either in front of or behind the anterior corneal surface.

A simpler modification that also allows the practitioner to ensure that the slit beam is normal to the cornea is to place above the slit aperture of the pachometer a small piece of translucent material. When the incident light is normal to the cornea, an image of the slit, after reflection at the cornea, will be seen on this material. While this modification is simpler than that of Mishima and Hedbys (1968), it does require the optometrist to take his or her eye away from the eyepiece in order to check normality of the incident beam.

   Another modification to the Haag–Streit pachometer has been made by Mandell and Polse (1969) who supplemented the simple scale fixed to the rotatable glass plate with an electronic transducer. This technique has been further developed and the results from the transducer can now be fed into a small computer which gives the mean and standard deviation of a series of measurements taken in quick succession. By taking a series of measurements in this way, the confidence that can be applied to the final result is improved.

   Ruben (1974) has suggested that the pachometer device can also be used to measure the thickness of soft contact lenses. The contact lens is placed over an acrylic sphere which is attached to the head rest of the slit lamp. Because the scale of the pachometer has been based upon the cornea's refractive index of 1.376, the results of such a measurement will have to be multiplied by the factor

$$\frac{CL^2 - 0.413}{1.2166}$$

where CL equals the refractive index of the lens (Donaldson, 1966).

Fundus examination

Slit lamps can also be used, with the addition of a lens between the microscope and the eye, to view the fundus. It is a particularly valuable technique because the binocular microscope provides a stereoscopic image

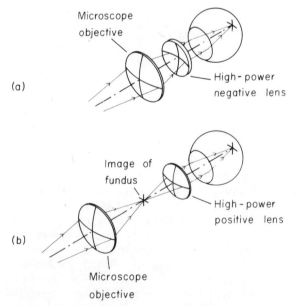

Figure 6.13. Fundus examination with a slit lamp: (a) with the aid of a negatively powered lens; (b) with the aid of a positively powered lens

of the retina that allows the practitioner to assess the depth of any optic nerve head cupping. Slit lamps cannot normally be focused any deeper into the eye than the anterior vitreous due to the refracting power of the cornea and lens. This problem can be overcome by one of two techniques. The first is to neutralize the power of the cornea with a high-power negative lens (*see Figure 6.13*(a)). The second is to use a high-power positive lens to form an intermediate image of the fundus at the focal plane of the microscope (*see Figure 6.13*(b)). Both techniques can be used either with lenses placed just in front of the eye or with contact lenses.

Of the non-contact lens techniques, the negatively powered Hruby lens is the most popular. When coupled with the microscope, so that lateral and vertical movements occur together, an area of retina of up to 30 degrees from the line of sight can be viewed. While uncoupling the microscope and lens allows an examination of a slightly larger area, it is considerably more clumsy. The use of non-contact positive lenses, such as the Bayadi lens, results in an inverted image and a longer working distance that may, with some slit lamps, be difficult to obtain. However, positive lenses give a slightly larger field of view and can be used successfully on high myopes whose fundi may not be visible with a Hruby lens. A disadvantage of positive lenses is that they give a large curvature of field (Schmidt, 1975).

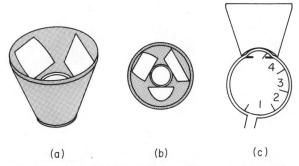

(a)   (b)   (c)

Figure 6.14. (a) and (b) The Goldmann three-mirror lens for the examination of the fundus with a slit lamp. (c) The four regions of the retina visable through 1, the centre, and 2, 3 and 4, the three mirrors of the Goldmann lens

Of the contact lens devices, negative lenses are again by far the most popular. They usually have a cone-like extension from the edge of the lens that stops the patient from blinking, which reduces the optical quality of the lenses' front surface. These lenses allow the practitioner to directly view up to 30 degrees from the patient's line of sight. By using a lens that incorporates a mirror, such as the Goldmann three-mirror lens, the practitioner is able to view the whole of the patient's fundus. In this situation, the illuminating and viewing axes are directed towards a mirror that reflects them towards a peripheral region of the retina. The mirrors in the Goldmann three-mirror lens are set at slightly different angles such that, by successively viewing through each of them, the total retina can be examined (*see Figure 6.14*). The lens is rotated while on the eye in order to

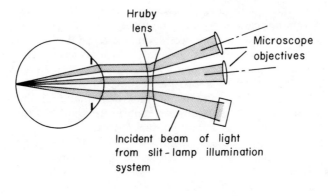

Position of illuminating beam and viewing paths within the patient's pupil

Figure 6.15. The position of the illuminating and viewing paths in the plane of the cornea

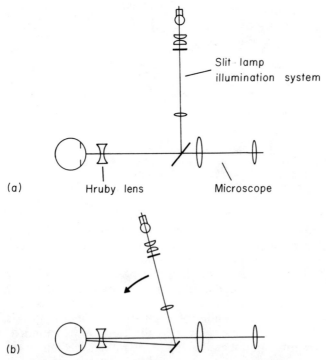

Figure 6.16. (a) The normal position of the slit illuminator. (b) The slit illuminator rotated so that its beam passes beneath the viewing paths at the plane of the pupil

direct the illumination and viewing axes towards the region of the retina that clinician wishes to examine.

For a clear, unhindered view of the fundus, it is essential that the cornea does not reflect any of the incident light into the viewing system. This can be achieved by positioning the light source such that there is no overlap, at the cornea, between the viewing and illuminating systems (*see Figure 6.15*). While this situation is not difficult to achieve while the practitioner is viewing the posterior pole of the eye, it can become a problem when he or she tries to view the periphery along the horizontal meridian (Tate and Safir, 1979). In this situation, the effective horizontal dimension of the pupil is reduced. Haag–Streit have incorporated a modification to their slit

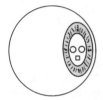

Position of the illuminating
and viewing paths

Figure 6.17. The horizontal dimension of the pupil decreases with oblique gaze. Vertical rotation of the slit axis allows the illuminating path to pass beneath the viewing paths

lamp that helps alleviate this problem. By tilting the light source about a horizontal axis and by changing the mirror, they have made it possible to place the path of the illuminating system below that of the viewing system (*see Figure 6.16*). With this arrangement, an unhindered view of the fundus can be obtained with a pupil of much smaller horizontal dimension (*see Figure 6.17*).

Gonioscopy

Gonioscopy is the technique used to see into the angle of the anterior chamber. It is important in the diagnosis of close-angle glaucoma and in the detection of certain iris pathologies. A direct view of the angle of the anterior chamber is not normally possible with the slit lamp because of the overhang of the opaque scleral shelf and the fact that light which emanates from the angle is reflected back into the eye by the cornea. This problem can be overcome with a contact lens that incorporates a mirror, such as the Goldmann single-mirror goniolens. The contact lens neutralizes the power of the cornea and the mirror reflects the illuminating and viewing axes of the slit lamp into the angle of the anterior chamber*. The Goldmann single-mirror lens has to be rotated in order to see all of the angle.

While initial examination is normally conducted with diffuse illumination, the optical section available with a narrow slit is also valuable in

* Goniscopy can be performed without a slit lamp: for a review of alternative techniques, the reader is referred to Becker (1972).

estimating the width of the angle. The slit image of the projection system has to be able to rotate in order for the optical section to be seen in meridians other than the vertical.

Tonometry

The Goldmann tonometer utilizes a slit lamp to both illuminate the eye and to make the applanated area visible to the examiner. The slit lamp's joystick arrangement is used to bring the tonometer head into gentle contact with the eye. For a more detailed description of this attachment, the reader is referred to chapter 3.

Laser photocoagulation

The technique of laser photocoagulation of the eye is often carried out with a slit lamp (Little, 1973)*. The output from a laser is combined with the illuminating source of the slit lamp by either a fibre optic or a series of connecting tubes. The ophthalmologist views the fundus through a contact lens (in the manner described in the section on fundus examination) and places the laser beam over the region of the retina in which a lesion is to be created. For alignment purposes, the laser light is filtered down to such an extent that it does not burn the retina, but remains visible to the ophthalmologist. Once in position, the laser system is triggered to produce a high intensity, brief pulse of light that can create the required lesion.

   Precise manipulation of the laser beam is made possible by a series of optical elements added to the slit lamp's illumination system, which allow the laser beam to be moved around independently of the slit illumination beam. A description of the specific forms of treatment and the pathologies amenable to photocoagulation can be found in Morse (1979).

Attachment for measuring visual acuity in patients with hazy media

When a cataract is removed from a patient's eye, the ophthalmologist often has no knowledge as to what the final visual acuity of the patient will be because the cataract has prevented the patient's fundus from being viewed. The ophthalmologist, therefore, does not know if the retina has deteriorated during the time that the cataract has been present. Rodenstock have recently developed an attachment to the slit lamp that allows the ophthalmologist to estimate the patient's retinal acuity while the cataract is still present. This attachment is based upon a technique first described by Campbell and Green (1965) and later applied to the cataractous eye by Goldmann (1972) and Green (1970). In the Rodenstock instrument a laser is utilized to produce two coherent beams of light that, when passed into the eye, form an interference pattern at the retina (*see Figure 6.18*). The

---

* It can also be carried out with an indirect ophthalmoscope.

interference pattern appears as a grating of black and red lines. The visual acuity of the patient is measured by altering the spatial frequency of the grating, the finest resolvable grating being taken as a measure of the patient's retinal acuity. Rodenstock have calibrated the instrument on normal subjects such that a given grating acuity can be converted into an equivalent Snellen fraction.

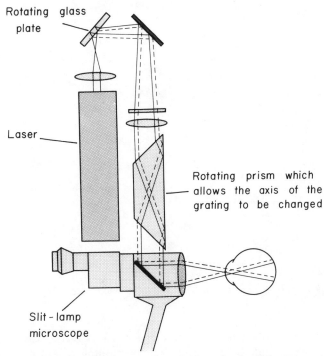

Rotating glass plate

Laser

Rotating prism which allows the axis of the grating to be changed

Slit-lamp microscope

Figure 6.18. Laser acuity measuring attachment for the slit lamp (Rodenstock)

The two coherent beams of light are brought to focus at separate points in or near the entrance pupil of the eye. The frequency of the grating formed on the retina is dependent upon the separation of the two beams in the pupil and the wavelength of the laser light. It is by decreasing or increasing the separation of the beams that the frequency of the grating is changed. The ability of a cataractous patient to see the grating is dependent upon the ophthalmologist finding two relatively clear points in the lens through which to shine the laser light. If two points cannot be found, then a reliable measure of the retinal acuity cannot be made. The value of the slit lamp in this procedure is to provide the opthalmologist with a means of viewing and adjusting the points where the laser light passes through the pupil.

Lotmar (1980) has described a similar attachment to a Haag–Streit slit lamp (*see Figure 6.19*). Instead of using a laser interference pattern to bypass the optics of the eye, it uses what is, in effect, a very small pin hole.

The pin hole is imaged in the plane of the pupil where its size is only 0.2 mm. The target used in the Haag–Streit instrument is composed of two gratings, which can be rotated with respect to each other, to form a Moiré fringe at the patient's retina. This system, which according to Lotmar (1980) gives comparable results to the interference technique, has the advantages of only requiring a single clear point within the lens and of being operable with light of any wavelength.

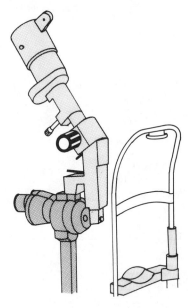

Figure 6.19. Lotmar's acuity measuring attachment to the Haag–Streit slit lamp

The drawback with both these techniques is that while a positive result tells the ophthalmologist that the retina is still functioning correctly, a negative result does not necessarily mean that the retina is damaged. It may merely mean that the ophthalmologist has not found a clear region within the lens through which to pass the light.

References

BECKER, S. C. (1972). *Clinical Gonioscopy.* Mosby, St. Louis
BEDWELL, C. H. (1978). The Diag slit lamp binocular microscope. *Optician*, **175**, Jan 27th, 17
CAMPBELL, F. W. and GREEN, D. G. (1965). Optical and retinal factors affecting visual resolution. *Journal of Physiology*, **181**, 576
DAVEY, J. (1977). Experiences with the Zeiss 10SL slit lamp. *Ophthalmic Optician*, **17**, April 16th, 328
DONALDSON, D. D. (1966). A new instrument for the measurement of cornea thickness. *Archives of Ophthalmology*, **76**, 25
EHLERS, N. and KRUSE HANSEN, F. (1971). On the optical measurement of corneal thickness. *Acta Ophthalmologica*, **49**, 65
GOLDMANN, H. (1972). Examination of the fundus of the cataractous eye. *American Journal of Ophthalmology.* **73**, 309
GREEN, D. G. (1970). Testing the vision of cataractous patients by means of laser generated interference fringes. *Science*, **168**, 1240

JUILLERAT and KOBY, F. E. (1928), cited in Ehlers and Kruse Hansen (1971)

LITTLE, H. (1973). Argon laser retinal photocoagulation: Instrumentation and general techniques. In *Documentum Ophthalmologica Proceedings Series, Symposium on Light Coagulation* Vol. 1, p. 17. Edited by J. Francois,

LITTMANN, H (1950). A new slit lamp apparatus. *American Journal of Ophthalmology*, **33,** 1863

LOTMAR, W. (1980). Apparatus for the measurement of retinal visual acuity by Moire fringes. *Investigative Ophthalmology*, **19,** 393

MANDELL, R. B. and POLSE, K. A. (1969). Keratoconus: Spatial variation of corneal thickness is a diagnostic test. *Archives of Ophthalmology*, **82,** 182

MISHIMA, S. and HEDBYS, B. O. (1968). Measurement of cornea thickness with the Haag–Streit pachometer. *Archives of Ophthalmology*, **80,** 710

MORSE, P. H. (1979). Photocoagulation. In *Clinical Ophthalmology*, Vol. 5, Ch. 19, p. 1. Edited by T. D. Duane. Harper and Row, Hagerstown

RUBEN, M. (1974). Soft lenses: The physico-chemical characteristics. *Contacto*, **18,** 11

SASIENI, L. S. (1981). A guide to slit lamps. *Optician*, **181,** 40

SCHMIDT, T. A. F. (1975). On slit lamp microscopy. *Documenta Ophthalmologica*, **39,** 117

TATE, G. W. and SAFIR, A. (1979). The slit lamp. In *Clinical Ophthalmology*, Vol. 1, Ch. 59, p. 1. Edited by T. D. Duane. Harper and Row, Hagerstown

7

Ophthalmic photography

The practice of ophthalmic photography is still largely confined to institutions where the photographs are used for educational purposes and to document and monitor specific eye conditions. No one doubts the immense value that photographs have in the training of new clinicians. Recently, however, several articles have appeared within the literature that encourage the practitioner to undertake ophthalmic photography. These articles point out that photography is now much easier and cheaper to perform and that photographs can be valuable not only in the ways the institutions use them, but also in the explanation of a condition to a patient and in the referral of a patient.

Within this chapter I have divided ophthalmic photography into four groups:

1. External eye photography;
2. Slit lamp photography;
3. Fundus photography;
4. Photography of the corneal endothelium.

The last three groups all require specialist equipment, which is normally provided with detailed instructions on how to obtain good photographs. External eye photography, however, is usually carried out with standard camera equipment, which is not provided with instructions on how to take photographs of the external eye. I will therefore include in this section the recommended procedures for external eye photography as outlined by Bishop (1976), Burns (1980), Long (1979) and Olsen (1979).

External eye photography

External eye photography covers everything from a full-face portrait to a close up of one eye. It does not require expensive equipment and much, if not all, of the equipment can be used for other types of photography.

Camera

The best type of camera for photographing the external eye is known as a single lens reflex (SLR). With this type of camera, the photographer views through the main lens of the camera and thus sees exactly what will be photographed. Cameras with separate viewfinders have small parallax errors which become significant when close-up photographs are taken. While almost any type of SLR camera can be used, care should be taken to choose one that has a viewfinder screen that allows critical focusing. Certain cameras, such as those made by Nikon and Canon, allow different types of viewfinder screens to be fitted. Olsen (1979) recommends the type of screen that has a clear central area with cross hairs, surrounded by a ground glass area. This type of viewfinder allows better focusing at high magnification than does the more commonly found type, which has a split image rangefinder with microprism. Another major advantage of the SLR cameras is that they invariably allow different types of lenses to be fitted, which, as you will see from the next section, allows the photographer to select the most appropriate type.

Lens

The type of lens system required is dependent upon three factors:

1. The type of photograph requried (i.e. what magnification is necessary);
2. The cost;
3. The photographic equipment already available.

Table 7.1 shows the magnification required for different types of photograph. A magnification of ×1 means that 35 mm in the object plane will fill a 35 mm frame, while a magnification of ×0.5 means that 70 mm in the object plane will fill a 35 mm frame.

TABLE 7.1. The magnification required for different types of external eye photographs

Subject	Magnification
Single eye	×1
Eye and orbit	×0.5
Both eyes	×0.25–0.3
Full-face portrait	×0.1–0.2

If you are buying a camera for the first time, then the best type of lens to purchase with it is a 50 or 55 mm macrolens. This type of lens allows you to focus on objects much closer to the camera than is normally possible with a standard 50 or 55 mm lens. By decreasing the distance between the subject and the camera lens, the higher magnifications required for external ophthalmic photography are obtained. When going out to buy a camera, you can usually ask your dealer to provide the camera with a 50 or 55 mm macrolens, rather than the standard 50 or 55 mm lens, for only a minor increase in expenditure. Most macrolenses allow magnifications of up to ×0.5. Higher magnifications can be achieved with the same lens when it is used with any one of the following four accessories:

1. Extension tubes;
2. A bellows unit;
3. Close-up lenses;
4. A teleconverter.

Extension tubes

Extension tubes are simple hollow tubes that are placed between the camera lens and the camera body (*see Figure 7.1*(b)). By increasing the distance between the lens and the film plane they allow shorter subject-to-lens distances and thus higher magnifications.

Bellows units

Bellows units are also placed between the camera lens and the camera body and operate in exactly the same way as extension tubes. They are slightly more convenient to use than extension tubes in that the extent of the extension can be changed without having to remove the lens.

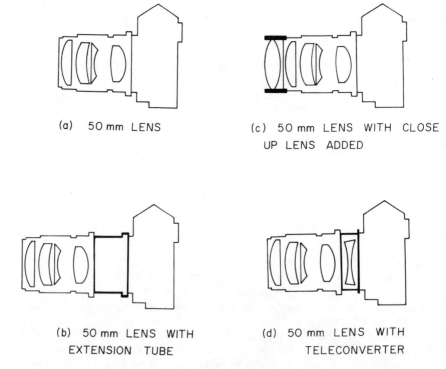

(a)   50 mm LENS

(c) 50 mm LENS WITH CLOSE UP LENS ADDED

(b) 50 mm LENS WITH EXTENSION TUBE

(d) 50 mm LENS WITH TELECONVERTER

Figure 7.1. Four techniques of increasing the magnification of a single lens reflex camera

Close-up lenses

Close-up lenses are simple positive lenses that fit in front of the existing camera lens (*see Figure 7.1*(c)). They increase the effective power of the camera lens and thereby allow it to be focused on objects much closer to the lens. A disadvantage of close-up lenses, which normally range in power from 1 D to 10 D, is that their optics are usually of poor quality. Photographs taken with these lenses, particularly the ones of higher power, have a slight fuzziness which is most evident at the edge of the photograph. A further disadvantage of these lenses is that, for a given amount of magnification, they require a shorter working distance than would be required with extension tubes or bellows units (Olsen, 1979). As the working distance becomes shorter, it becomes increasingly difficult for the flash gun to evenly illuminate the subject.

Teleconverters

Teleconverters receive a mixed response from photographers. Those in favour say it is a simple and cheap way of increasing the magnification, while those against say it drastically reduces the quality of the image. A teleconverter fits between the camera lens and the camera body in the same place as the extension tubes (*see Figure 7.1*(d)). It contains a negative lens which effectively increases the focal length of the camera lens. By operating in this manner, it does not require the short working distances that are often a problem with close-up lenses. The use of teleconverters has been described by Long (1979).

If you already have an SLR camera with a standard 50 or 55 mm lens and are unwilling to purchase a new lens, then the magnifications required for external eye photography can still be achieved with any one of the four techniques just outlined. However, because the standard 50 or 55 mm lenses are not designed to be used for close-up work, they tend, when used in this way, to have more aberrations than macrolenses and therefore produce photographs of slightly inferior quality.

If you do not have an SLR camera, but have a camera with a fixed lens and a viewfinder, and you still want to do some external eye photography, then this can be achieved with the use of close-up lenses. If you set your camera for infinity and place a +5.00 D close-up lens in front of it, then you should be in focus for objects 20 cm in front of the close-up lens. If you propose to use this technique, then it is advisable to build an extension bar to the close-up lens that positions the lens at exactly the right distance from the patient's face.

Illumination system

In order to illuminate the eye sufficiently for external eye photography, a flash attachment has to be used. No special type of flash gun is required. The more expensive automatic (light feedback regulated) flashes are of no advantage because, for the short working distances used, manual setting is recommended (Olsen, 1979). The normal positioning of a flash gun, on the top of the camara body (*see Figure 7.2*(a)), is not suitable for external eye photography for three reasons. First, the flash points in the wrong direction for close-up photographs, which means that a lot of light is unnecessarily wasted. Second, the lens, especially if it has several extension tubes attached to it, may create a shadow over the subject. Finally, the normal position does not allow the photographer to control the position of the corneal reflex. This reflex, which appears on the photograph as an image of the flash gun, is produced by the cornea reflecting a proportion of the incident light. On occasions this reflex can obscure the subject of the photograph.

Position of flash gun for normal photography

Recommended position of flash gun for external eye photography

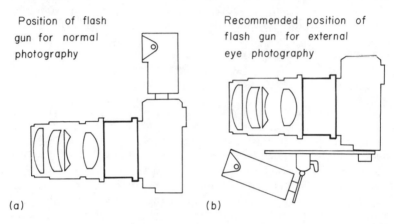

(a)   (b)

Figure 7.2. Position of the flash gun for external eye photography

To overcome these problems, a straight flash bracket with a universal swivel arm should be used. The straight bracket will allow the flash gun to be attached underneath the lens (*see Figure 7.2*(b)), or to either side of it, thereby offering the photographer control over the positioning of the reflex. The swivel arm, which attaches to the end of the bracket, allows the flash gun to be pointed at the subject.

To establish where the corneal reflex will appear on the photograph a small light source, such as a hand-held slit lamp, can be attached to the flash gun when setting up the equipment. The reflex of this light source will appear at roughly the same position as the flash gun reflex in the final photograph.

It is possible to buy a special type of flash gun known as a ring flash that, as the name suggests, is ring shaped and fits snugly around the camera lens. This type of flash gun is not of great value for photographs of the eye for two reasons. First, it produces a shadowless light which obscures surface irregularities which may very well be the subject of the photograph. Second, the positioning of the corneal reflex cannot be controlled (Mandell, Foster and Luther, 1976).

While the flash gun provides the illumination for the photograph, a second source of illumination is necessary for focusing the camera. A standard anglepoise lamp directed towards the patient's eye is ideal for this purpose.

Setting up

While not being absolutely necessary, it is certainly a great help to have the patient's head stabilized with a head rest and to have the camera mounted on a small tripod (*see Figure 7.3*). This arrangement, which fixes the

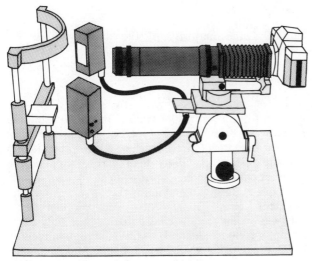

Figure 7.3. Anterior segment camera (Nikon)

distance between the camera and the patient, enables the practitioner to more accurately focus the camera. Rather than buy a head rest solely for this purpose, it is often possible to use one that is attached to some other piece of equipment such as a keratometer or slit lamp.

Exposure

Guide numbers for different speeds of film are given with the flash gun. In theory, the guide number divided by the distance (in ft) from the camera to the subject should give you the correct exposure, e.g. with a guide number of 45 and a subject at 10 ft, an exposure of $f/4.5$ is recommended. Unfortunately, for working distances of under 1 m this relationship no longer holds.

Gutner (1977) recommends that the exposure be based upon the magnification used, the exposure being $f/32$ for magnifications of ×1, ×0.5 and ×0.33 and $f/22$ for magnifications of ×0.25 and ×0.2. These values are for a flash gun the guide number of which is 40–44 with a film speed of 25 ASA. If a flash gun with a different guide number or a film with a different speed is used, then the new exposure can be calculated from equation (7.1)

$$\text{new } f/\text{number} = \frac{f/\text{number recommended by Gutner} \times \text{guide number for film used}}{42} \quad (7.1)$$

The exposure calculated in this way is only a guide. It is wise to take at least three photographs, one at the calculated f/number, one at the next higher f/number and one at the next lower f/number. The shutter speed for flash photography should be set to synchronize with the flash (usually 1/60th second).

Film

The films recommended by the majority of the authors cited are Kodachrome 25 (25 ASA) and Kodachrome 64 (64 ASA).

Fluorescein photography of the external eye

Two types of external eye photograph frequently required by the optometrist are a fluorescein fit of a contact lens and a fluorescein staining of the cornea. If the practitioner attempts to photograph fluorescein stain with the techniques just described the contrast between the fluorescein and the eye will be low and as a result the subject of the photograph will be poorly defined. The contrast can be increased with the aid of two filters. The first is placed in front of the flash gun and limits the wavelength of the incident light to that which 'excites' fluorescence. The second (barrier filter) is placed in front of the camera lens where it transmits only those wavelengths that arise from the fluorescence. The filters recommended by Bishop (1976) are the Wratten 48 as an excitor and the Kodak colour-compensating filter No. cc 50Y as the barrier filter. Gutner (1979) recommends two slightly different filters, the Wratten 47A as an excitor and the Nikon Y48 as a barrier. Gutner also states that the aperture of the lens should be increased by 3.5 stops to compensate for the loss of light through the filters. As you will appreciate, this increase in aperture will result in a considerable loss in depth of field and a consequent sensitivity to slight focus errors. Those who wish to take fluorescein photographs should not, therefore, choose a low cost system, but should purchase the more expensive macrolenses.

Special systems for external eye photography

Rodenstock produce a camera system for photographing the external eye that attaches to their 2000 series slit lamp. The camera is attached to the top of the microscope body and views the eye through a narrow prism placed between the microscope objectives. The camera's focus is set to coincide with that of the microscope which means that the operator merely has to focus the microscope on the subject in order to focus the camera.

The flash gun is attached to the slit illumination system via a mechanical coupling that allows the flash gun to be raised or lowered with respect to the slit illuminator. This freedom of movement combined with that of the slit illuminator means that the flash gun can be positioned in such a way as to place the corneal reflex of the flash away from the subject of the photograph. The two major advantages of this system are, first, that the slit lamp's own illumination system can be used to accurately focus the microscope and camera, and second, that the chin rest helps the patient to keep his head steady during the photograph.

Even though the slit illumination system may be on during the photograph, the optical section it produces will not be seen in the final photograph due to the relative brightness of the diffuse flash. A disadvantage of the Rodenstock system is that it cannot be used to take either full-face or half-face portraits.

Recently, Nikon have produced an anterior segment camera unit which contains a camera with close-up lens, a pair of flash guns mounted on flexible arms and a chin rest (*see Figure 7.3*). As the camera and chin rest are mounted on an ophthalmic instrument table, they can be ready to take a photograph whenever the practitioner desires. Unlike the Rodenstock instrument, the unit does not have the advantage of a separate illumination system to precisely focus the camera.

Slit lamp photography

Slit lamp cameras (*Figure 7.4*) enable the practitioner to photograph the anterior segment of the eye and the fundus as seen with the slit lamp (*see* Chapter 6). Slit lamp cameras can be divided into two groups:

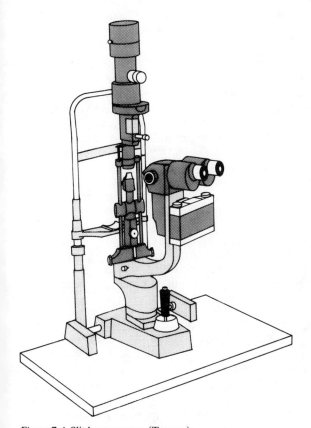

Figure 7.4. Slit lamp camera (Topcon)

1. Those that view through the eyepeice of the slit lamp's microscope and use the existing slit illumination;
2. Those that incorporate a flash unit within the slit illumination system that increases the intensity of the slit.

Slit lamp cameras that view through the eyepiece

It is possible to purchase a connector which will attach almost any camera to the eyepiece of a slit lamp. With the eyepiece focus adjuster set at zero and the camera set for infinity, the same image as that normally seen by the practitioner will be formed at the film plane of the camera (Zantos and Pye, 1979).

The problem with the system is that of providing sufficient light from the standard slit illuminator to create a sufficiently bright image. It is usually necessary to set the aperture of the camera at the maximum value, to have the slit as bright as possible and to make the exposure time long. Unfortunately, this results in excessive patient lacrimation due to the bright light, a poor depth of field and a likelihood of eye movements blurring the image (Gutner, 1979). The technique has, however, been successfully used by Zantos and Holden (1977) to photograph the corneal endothelium (*see* section on corneal endothelium photography, p. 148.

Slit lamp cameras with built-in flash units

Instruments with built-in units are much more expensive and sophisticated than those described in the previous section. They incorporate a flash gun within the slit lamp's illumination system which, when triggered, brings the intensity of the slit up to a very high level. This high intensity means that the aperture of the camera system can be set below that required of the instruments that view through the eyepiece and that the shutter speed can be increased. These two factors will improve the quality of image by increasing its depth of field and by being less sensitive to eye and head movements. Although the flash intensity is very bright, its short duration means that it does not cause any discomfort to the patient or damage to the eye.

Cameras for this type of instrument are usually attached to the microscope body and view through one of the microscope's objectives via a beam splitter (Zeiss (Oberkochen)) or a reflex mirror which flips into the observation system when the photograph is being taken. This arrangement allows the practitioner to view the section of the eye to be photographed up until the instant that the photograph is taken. Because the number of optical elements between the film plane and the eye are reduced with this system (in comparison with those described above), the optical quality of the image is again improved. The focus of these cameras is set to coincide with that of the microscope.

The majority of slit lamp cameras that fall into this category have a second low-power flash system that provides fill-in to the photograph. Without this the photographs tend to look rather spartan, showing literally just a section through the eye within a sea of darkness. The fill-in flash provides sufficient background illumination for the rest of the eye to be seen in the photograph without significantly affecting the image of the slit.

With some of the slit lamp cameras it is possible to obtain stereophotographs of the eye. These are particularly valuable when viewing the disc as they provide the practitioner with an estimation of the depth of any cupping.

Fundus photography

Fundus cameras are optically based upon Gullstrand's reflex free ophthalmoscope (*see* Chapter 1 and *Figure 1.5*). The exit pupil of the illumination system and the entrance pupil of the viewing system are both imaged in separate regions of the pupil. This arrangement ensures that the reflections of the light source from both the cornea and lens do not enter the viewing system. Fundus cameras contain two light sources. The first, a tungsten filament source, is used to illuminate the fundus while the operator focuses and aligns the camera. It is the same type of light source as that found in other indirect ophthalmoscopes. The second source is a flash which momentarily increases the illumination of the fundus to a level that can be recorded with a camera.

Both these light sources need to operate through the normal illumination system of the ophthalmoscope to ensure that the image is reflex free. This is achieved by one of the following three techniques:

1. A swing away mirror;
2. A semi-transparent mirror;
3. By transillumination.

The swing away mirror

This is the simplest technique. It consists of a simple mirror that, under normal viewing conditions, reflects the light from the viewing source and occludes the flash lamp (*see Figure 7.5*). Just before the photograph is taken, the mirror flips out of the way of the flash lamp, thereby allowing its light to reach the fundus.

Semi-transparent mirror

With this technique a semi-transparent mirror reflects a proportion of the light from the viewing source and transmits a proportion of the light from the flash source (*see Figure 7.5*). It has the advantage over the first technique that it does not require any moving parts, but has the disadvantage that it requires higher intensity sources because of the loss of light incurred by either reflection or transmission through the semi-transparent mirror.

Transillumination

This technique involves no moving parts and yet allows the full intensities of both sources to reach the fundus. To enable this, the viewing lamp is imaged by a condenser within the helix of the flash source (*see Figure 7.5*). This image has the character of a 'quasi-source' located in exactly the same position as the flash source. In the observation system, a reflex mirror is normally used to reflect the light towards the observer's eyepiece. This mirror flips out of the way during a photograph to allow the light to reach the film plane.

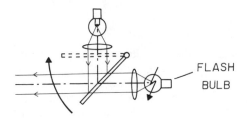

FLASH
BULB

SWING   AWAY   MIRROR

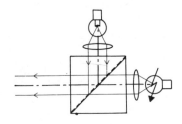

SEMI-TRANSPARENT   MIRROR

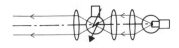

TRANSILLUMINATION

Figure 7.5. Three different types of illumination systems found in fundus cameras

The field of view of most fundus cameras is 30 degrees which means that they are capable of photographing, within a single frame, an area that extends from the nasal side of the optic disc to the temporal side of the macula. Canon and Nikon have both recently designed fundus cameras with 45 degree fields of view. Leutwein and Littmann (1979) have, however, pointed out that the oblique astigmatism and curvature of field at the periphery of the retina means that the image quality of cameras with large fields of view must be expected to deteriorate towards the periphery of the field. The same problem arises when cameras with 30 degree fields are used to photograph the periphery of the fundus.

Busse and Mittelman (1976) have calculated that between 10 and 15 D of oblique astigmatism will be produced when the light that strikes the refracting surfaces of the eye is at 30 degrees to the eye's optical axis. They have developed a modification to the Zeiss (Oberkochen) fundus camera that allows this astigmatism to be neutralized by a variable astigmatic element within the camera. The improvement in the quality of the images is spectacular. The system can also be used to correct refractive astigmatic errors, thereby improving the quality of photographs taken along the optical axis of astigmatic eyes. A similar astigmatic lens is offered as an accessory to the Nikon fundus camera.

Pomerantzeff (1971) has described a fundus camera known as the 'equator plus camera' that has a 148 degree field of view when measured from the nodal point of the patient's eye. This large field of view is obtained by having the objective lens of the camera in contact with the cornea. The camera illuminates the fundus via two rings of fibre optic bundles that shine through the periphery of the cornea. This type of illumination system requires a pupil diameter of about 8 mm in order to illuminate the whole fundus. When it is not possible to get such a large pupil, equator plus photography can still be performed with transcleral illumination.

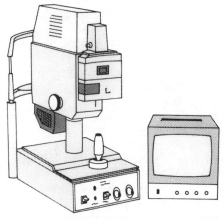

Figure 7.6. Non mydriatic fundus camera (Canon)

Normal fundus cameras require a pupil diameter of 4–5 mm. This size of pupil cannot normally be obtained while the fundus is being viewed without the aid of a mydriatic. To overcome the need for a mydriatic, Canon and Topcon have recently produced fundus cameras where the illumination of the viewing system is provided by a low-power infra-red light (*see Figure 7.6*). This light source is invisible to the patient and therefore does not produce any miosis. The infra-red light reflected from the fundus is imaged on a special TV tube which relays this image to a nearby monitor. The flash guns within these cameras use visible light. Their speed, however, is so fast that the pupil does not have time to react before the photograph is taken.

Over the years, fundus cameras have become an integral part of the technique of fluorescein angiography. The passage of dye through the fundus circulation occurs so quickly that a thorough analysis of it can only be made from a series of photographs taken at a rate of approximately 3–4 per second. In addition to a special film-advance mechanism and a special power supply, the fundus cameras used for fluorescein angiography require two optical filters. The first, an excitor filter, is placed within the illuminating system and limits the wavelengths that enter the eye to those that excite fluorescence. The second, a barrier filter, is placed within the viewing system and limits the wavelengths that reach the film plane to those which come from the fluorescing dye. The combined effect of these filters is to increase the contrast of the fluorescein dye.

Photography of the corneal endothelium

A specialized form of photography that has recently received considerable interest in optometry due to its possible relevance to contact lens work is that of photographing the corneal endothelium (Zantos and Holden, 1977; Barr and Schoessler, 1980). There are two techniques currently used. The first was described by Brown (1970) and has been developed by Zantos and Holden (1977). It involves photographing the specular reflex of the endothelium produced by the illuminating system of a standard slit lamp. The problem of the reflex produced by the anterior surface of the iornea, which usually obscures the endothelium, is overcome by separating the illuminating and viewing systems by as large an angle as possible. In order to obtain high magnification, Zantos and Holden (1977) photographed the endothial reflex through the eyepiece of the slit lamp. The problem of insufficient illumination, normally experienced when attempting to photograph through the eyepeice, is not encountered with this technique because the specular reflex provides an extremely bright object.

The second technique involves the use of a specially designed instrument known as a specular microscope. The specular microscope was designed by Maurice (1968) and modified by Laing, Sandstron and Leibowitz (1975) to enable *in vivo* measurements. It has been further developed by Bourne (1976) to allow routine clinical measurements of the corneal endothelium. The objective, which has to make contact with the cornea, forms a slit image which measures some 100×400 microns at the endothelium. The illuminating and viewing systems are kept separate as they pass through the objective, in order to remove the reflex formed from the anterior corneal surface. The use of a narrow slit reduces the effect of scattered light from the stroma, but has a major disadvantage of only allowing a very small part of the endothelium to be photographed at any one time. Such a small area of endothelium makes it very difficult to conduct longitudinal studies due to the problem of locating the same part of the endothelium at each visit.

A modification to the standard specular microscope has been described by Koester, Campbell and Donn (1980). With the use of a scanning mirror, fields of 800 microns in diameter have been achieved with no loss in contrast. The technique allows continuous viewing of the 800 micron diameter area because of the high speed of mirror oscillation.

References

BARR, J. T. and SCHOESSLER, J. P. (1980). Corneal endothelia response to rigid contact lenses. *American Journal of Optometry and Physiological Optics*, **57**, 267

BISHOP, C. (1976). Basic aspects of ophthalmic photography. *Ophthalmic Optician,* **16,** 719, 762, 817, 845

BOURNE, B. M. (1976). Photography of the corneal endothelium. In *Ophthalmic Photography.* Edited by J. Justice. *International Ophthalmic Clinics,* **16(2),** 199

BROWN, N. (1970). Macrophotography of the anterior segment of the eye. *British Journal of Ophthalmology,* **54,** 697

BURNS, D. C. (1980). External eye photography. In *Contact Lenses,* 2nd Edn., Vol. 1, p. 155. Edited by J. S. Stone and A. J. Phillips. Butterworths, London

BUSSE, B. J. and MITTELMAN, D. (1976). Use of the astigmatism device on the Zeiss fundus camera for peripheral photography. In *Ophthalmic Photography.* Edited by J. Justice. *International Ophthalmic Clinics,* **16(2),** 63

GUTNER, R. K. (1977). Anterior segment photography. *Journal of the American Optometric Association,* **48,** 41

GUTNER, R. K. (1979). Slit lamp photodocumentation. *American Journal of Optometry and Physiological Optics,* **56,** 559

KOESTER, C. J., CAMPBELL, C. J. and DONN, A. (1980). Ophthalmic optical instruments: Two recent developments. *Japanese Journal of Ophthalmology,* **24,** 1

LAING, R. A., SANDSTRON, M. M. and LEIBOWITZ, H. M. (1975). In vivo photomicrography of the cornea endothelium. *Archives of Ophthalmology,* **93,** 143

LONG, W. F. (1979). A simple system for external ophthalmic photography. *Canadian Journal of Optometry,* **41,** 67

LEUTWEIN, K. and LITTMAN, H. (1979). The fundus camera. In *Clinical Ophthalmology,* Vol. 1, Ch. 61, p. 1. Edited by T. D. Duane. Harper and Row, Hagerstown

MANDELL, A. I., FOSTER, C. W. and LUTHER, J. D. (1976). External photography of the eye. In *Ophthalmic Photography.* Edited by J. Justice. *International Ophthalmic Clinics,* **16(2),** 133

MAURICE, D. M. (1968). Cellular membrane activity in the corneal endothelium of the intact eye. *Experientia,* **24,** 1094

OLSEN, O. J. (1979). External ophthalmic photography. *American Journal of Optometry and Physiological Optics,* **56,** 548

POMERANTZEFF, O. (1971). Equator-plus camera. *Investigative Ophthalmology,* **14,** 401

ZANTOS, S. G. and HOLDEN, B. A. (1977). Transient endothelial changes soon after wearing soft contact lenses. *American Journal of Optometry and Physiological Optics,* **54,** 856

ZANTOS, S. G. and PYE, D. C. (1979). Clinical photography in optometric practice. *Australian Journal of Optometry,* **67,** 279

8

Optometers

Optometers are devices for measuring the refractive state of the eye. They can be divided into two main groups, subjective and objective. Subjective optometers are those that use the criterion of blurredness or sharpness of a test object, while objective optometers contain an optical system which determines the vergence of light reflected from the patient's retina.

In this chapter, I first of all deal with two very basic subjective instruments. While these two instruments are now rarely, if ever, used to refract patients, they do demonstrate the principles upon which some of the more complex instruments are based. Following this, I describe the objective optometers that rely upon the operator to focus or align images formed upon the patient's retina. This is followed by a description of the infra-red optometers and, finally, two recently developed subjective instruments. It is hoped that by dealing with optometers in this order the reader will be able to see how some of the more complex instruments are based upon simple principles.

Two basic subjective instruments

The simple optometer

The simple optometer is a subjective instrument composed of a single optometer lens and a movable target (*see Figure 8.1*). The vergence of light

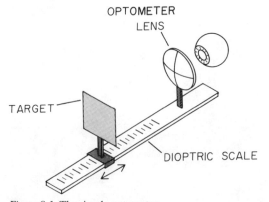

Figure 8.1. The simple optometer

from the target, after passing through the optometer lens, is dependent upon the position of the target (*see Figure 8.2*). An estimation of the patient's refraction is obtained by instructing the patient to move the target towards the optometer lens from a position of blurredness to one of sharpness. The point at which the target becomes sharp is taken as the measure of the refraction.

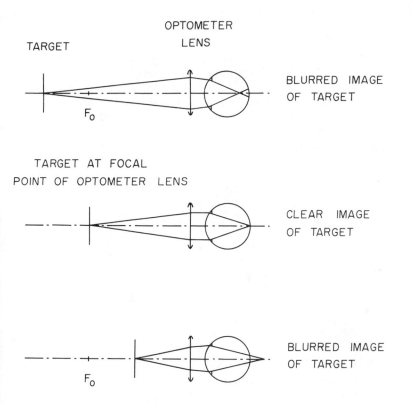

Figure 8.2. For an emmetropic patient the target is out of focus when it is not at the focal point of the optometer lens

The problems with this optometer are:

1. The patient nearly always accommodates due to the known proximity of the target;
2. Movement of the target beyond the point where it is first seen in focus stimulates the patient's accommodation;
3. The large depth of focus makes the setting inaccurate;
4. The scale is not linear;
5. The retinal image size of the target varies with its position from the optometer lens;
6. In its basic form, it cannot be used to measure astigmatic errors.

Two of these problems, namely the non-linear scale and the changing retinal image size with target position, can be overcome by placing the optometer lens such that its focal point coincides with either:

1.   The nodal point of the eye; or
2.   The anterior focal point of the eye; or
3.   The entrance pupil of the eye.

Such an instrument is known as a Badal optometer.

Young's optometer

Young's optometer is a simple optometer which uses the Scheiner's disc principle to refract the eye. The target for this type of optometer is usually a single point of light which is moved back and forth until it is seen singly by the observer (*see Figure 8.3*). When the target is not focused correctly upon the retina, it will be seen both out of focus and doubled (*see Figure 8.4*). The blurring of the points, however, will be minimal due to the pin hole effect of the Scheiner disc.

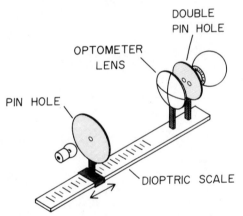

Figure 8.3. Young's optometer, which is based upon the Scheiner disc

Although the sensitivity of this type of optometer increases with the separation of the pin holes, even with the maximum separation it is not very high. In cases of astigmatism, the axis of the two points of light will not coincide with that of the pin holes except when the pin hole axis coincides with one of the astigmatic meridians. While in its basic form this optometer is rarely used to refract the eye, its principles are incorporated in both the Zeiss (Jena) refractometer (*see* pp. 158–162) and the 6600 Auto Refractor (*see* pp. 170–173).

Objective optometers

Introduction

Objective optometers rely upon the fact that some of the light incident upon the patient's retina will be diffusely reflected by the retinal surface.

An estimate of the refractive error can be made by either measuring the vergence of light that leaves the eye after reflection from the retina or by adjusting the vergence of light that enters the eye until a clear image of a target is formed on the retina's reflecting surface. The first approach is routinely used by optometrists when they perform retinoscopy. The second approach is used by the Rodenstock and Zeiss (Jena) optometers, both of which are discussed later on.

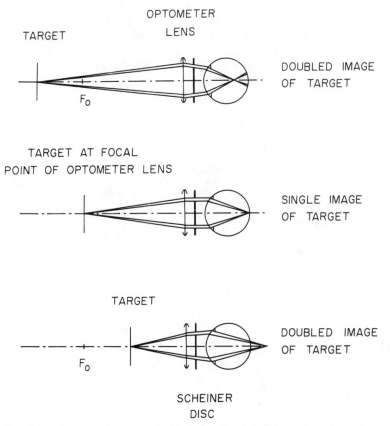

Figure 8.4. The patient's image is doubled when the pin hole target is not focused upon the retina

If the site of the reflecting layer does not coincide with the subjectively preferred focal plane, then an error will be introduced between the objective and subjective measures of the refraction. In the past, different layers in the retina have been proposed as the source of this reflex. Current data, however, indicate that several layers are jointly responsible and that the dominantly reflecting layer changes according to the wavelength of light used, whether the light is polarized or not, and the age of the patient (Charman and Jennings, 1976; Millodot and O'Leary, 1978; O'Leary and Millodot, 1978). To overcome this problem, the manufacturers of objective optometers calibrate their instruments with subjective measurements of the refraction. The dioptric scales of objective optometers are simply set to give, as near as possible, the same result as the subjective measurements.

The Astron refractometer

The Astron refractometer is a direct opthalmoscope which contains a movable target within its illuminating system (*see Figure 8.5*). Movement of the target, relative to the optometer lens, alters the vergence of light that enters the patient's eye. The optometrist views the image of the target formed upon the patient's retina through a lens which compensates both for the optometrist's refractive error and for that of the patient. The vergence of light that enters the patient's eye is adjusted until the target is judged to be in focus.

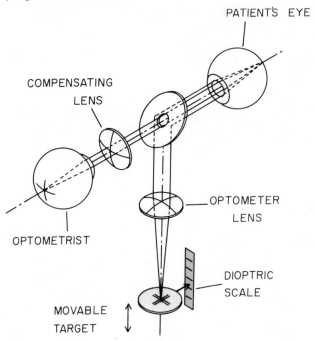

Figure 8.5. The Astron refractometer

In effect, the Astron refractometer can be considered as a simple optometer in which the optometrist, with the aid of a direct ophthalmoscope, makes the judgement of blurredness or sharpness rather than the patient.

The problems with this type of optometer are:

1. It is unable to measure cylindrical errors;
2. The intensity of the image is poor;
3. The corneal reflex is troublesome;
4. The depth of focus is large;
5. The patient tends to accommodate.

This tendency to accommodate arises from two sources. The first of these is that the patient knows the target is close to the eye. This knowledge results in a reflex accommodation known as proximal accommodation. The second source is due to the fact that the patient can see the target clearly when it is focused upon the retina. If the optometrist inadvertently moves the target too close to the optometer lens, then the patient will simply accommodate to keep it clear and the optometrist will continue to see a focused image upon the retina. Errors due to accommodation can be minimized if the optometrist adopts the recommended technique for the simple optometer – i.e. if the target is gradually brought towards the optometer lens from a position of blurredness until it just becomes clear.

The 'Projectoscope' made by Keeler is a type of Astron refractometer. This instrument (which is a modified specialist ophthalmoscope) should be positioned at the principle focus of the eye in order to be accurate. The accuracy of the Projectoscope is only of the order of ±1.00 D, but in fairness to Keeler it should be mentioned that this instrument was not designed as a refractometer, but as a device used for the treatment and diagnosis of certain binocular problems.

The Rodenstock refractometer

The Rodenstock refractometer (*see Figure 8.6*), unlike the Projectoscope, has been specifically designed to measure refractive errors. Its operating principles are basically the same as those of the Astron instrument in that it utilizes an ophthalmoscope to view the image of a target which is then focused upon the patient's retina. It differs from the Astron instrument by

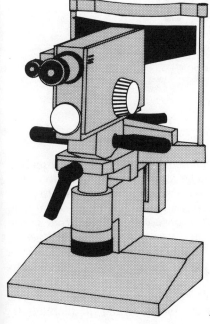

Figure 8.6. The Rodenstock PR 50 refractometer

using an indirect ophthalmoscope rather than a direct one. This modification allows the instrument to be reflex free (*see* p. 9). An isometric diagram of the optics of the Rodenstock instrument is given in *Figure 8.7*. The path length between the target and optometer lens is altered by moving a prism back and forth rather than by moving the target itself.

The observer compensates for his or her own refractive error in the Rodenstock instrument by adjusting the eyepiece until the stop S_1 is clearly in focus. After this adjustment, no further modification to the viewing

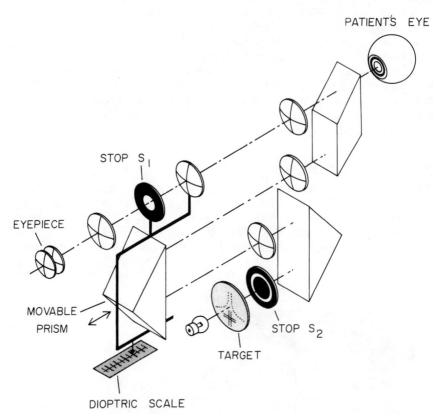

Figure 8.7. Optics of the Rodenstock PR 50 refractometer

system is necessary because of the mechanical coupling of the observing telescope to the prism adjuster. It should be recalled that in order to view a fundus clearly with a conventional ophthalmoscope, it is necessary to place a lens within the viewing system that compensates for the combined refractive error of the patient and the observer. In the Rodenstock instrument, the control that operates the prism and thus the vergence of light which enters the patient's eye, also adjusts the observing telescope such that when the target is focused on the retina, the retina is seen in focus through the telescope.

A complete ray diagram of the instrument is given in *Figure 8.8*. Points to notice are, first, that there is a stop, S_2, placed within the illuminating system which limits the light that enters the eye to an annulus and, second, that there is a stop, S_1, in the observation system which limits the observation system to the paraxial rays that return from the retina. Both these stops are imaged in the plane of the pupil, thereby making the instrument reflex free. By confining the measuring beam to the central region of the pupil, the manufacturers have increased the depth of focus of the instrument and thereby have made it more difficult for the operator to accurately focus the target.

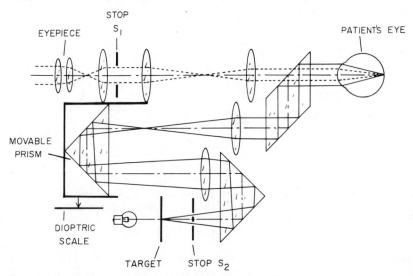

Figure 8.8. Ray diagram of the Rodenstock PR 50 refractometer

The target for the Rodenstock refractometer, which is capable of rotation around the optical axis of the refractometer, is shown in *Figure 8.9*. It is an opaque disc in which a series of holes and slits have been cut, which allow the passage of light from the source. It has been designed so as to be sensitive to astigmatic errors. The appearance of the target in cases of astigmatism is also shown in *Figure 8.9*. The axis of any astigmatism is read off directly from a scale attached to the target. The normal technique of measuring astigmatic errors with this instrument is to initially focus along the most positive meridian and then focus again along the most negative meridian. When the second measurement is taken, the patient can improve the image of the target by accommodating to bring the circle of least confusion closer to the retina. This accommodation will increase the amplitude of any measured astigmatism and therefore increase the error between the measured and the true refraction.

The Rodenstock instrument overcomes two of the problems of the Astron instrument; namely, the corneal reflex and the inability to measure astigmatic errors. The remaining problems are:

1. The intensity of the image is poor;
2. The patient tends to accommodate;
3. The depth of focus is large.

The instrument has been reviewed by both Bradford and Lawson (1954) and by Hobbs and Schimek (1956). Bradford and Lawson state that the instrument provides a relatively easy, rapid and accurate means of determining refractive error with cycloplaegia. Without cycloplaegia, they found the instrument less satisfactory due to accommodative problems.

Hobbs and Schimek (1956) also gave a generally favourable evaluation of the Rodenstock instrument. They claim that its chief disadvantage is the considerable degree of technical proficiency necessary to obtain accurate results. Inexperienced operators were found to have much greater problems with patient accommodation than did experienced operators.

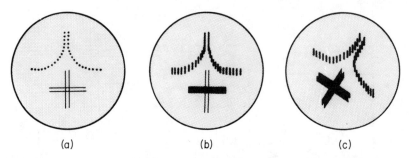

(a)   (b)   (c)

Figure 8.9. The target of the Rodenstock refractometer: (a) the target itself; (b) the appearance of the target in a case of astigmatism when the target is along one of the axes of astigmatism and the power is correctly set for one of the axes; (c) the appearance of the target when it is not along either of the axes of an astigmatic patient's eye

Volk (1955) compared the Rodenstock findings with those of retinoscopy and routine subjective procedures. He found that, on average, the retinoscope's findings were closer to the subjective ones than the Rodenstock's. From this he concluded that retinoscopy was more accurate than the Rodenstock instrument. He also found that the Rodenstock instrument had a mean error of -0.61 D in patients with active accommodation and -0.36 D in patients whose accommodation was paralyzed with a cycloplaegic. This finding indicates that the Rodenstock instrument stimulates the accommodative mechanism.

Hartinger coincidence optometer (Zeiss (Jena))

One of the major problems with the previously mentioned objective optometers is the inability to judge the exact point at which the target is correctly focused. The Hartinger coincidence optometer (*see Figure 8.10*) incorporates a modification that assists in making this judgement.

This modification consists of dividing the target into two and then passing the light from each half of the target through different parts of the pupil. If we consider, for the moment, that the target is composed of three vertical lines, as shown in *Figure 8.11*(a), then by passing the top half of the target through the left part of the pupil and the bottom half through the right, we can see that the retinal image will vary with the ametropia of the patient. In the case of myopia, the two half images will be displaced from each other, as shown in *Figure 8.11*(b), while in hyperopia, they will be

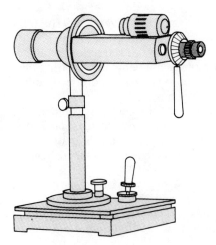

Figure 8.10. The Hartinger coincidence optometer (Zeiss (Jena))

TARGET

The light from the top half goes through the right side of the pupil. Light from the bottom half goes through the left side of the pupil

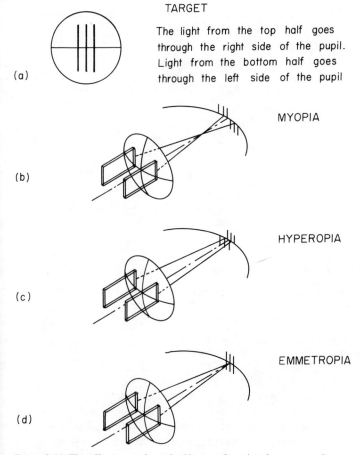

(a)

(b)   MYOPIA

(c)   HYPEROPIA

(d)   EMMETROPIA

Figure 8.11. The effect upon the retinal image of passing the upper and lower parts of a target through different parts of the pupil

displaced in the opposite direction, as shown in *Figure 8.11*(c). By adjusting the vergence of light that enters the eye, the two half images can be aligned (*see Figure 8.11*(d)), and a measure of the refraction obtained. Because the eye is capable of a much more accurate alignment setting than a judgment of focus, the accuracy of this optometer is theoretically much better than any of the instruments mentioned above.

The principle just described is similar to the Scheiner's disc principles of Young's optometer (*see* p. 152), only now the optometrist makes the judgment as to when the images are aligned, rather than the patient. As with the Scheiner disc, when the images are not aligned they are also out of focus.

On an astigmatic eye the displacement of the two half images will be oblique when the axes of the instrument and the astigmatism do not coincide (*see Figure 8.12*(a) and (b)). To be able to detect this situation and thus measure the axis of any astigmatism, two additional lines are placed

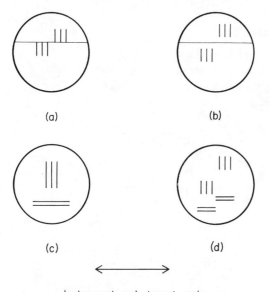

(a)

(b)

(c)

(d)

Instrument and target axis

Figure 8.12. Appearance of a target composed of three vertical lines when (a) there is a spherical error and (b) there is an astigmatic error, the axis of which does not coincide with that of the target. Appearance of the complete Zeiss target when (c) the instrument is at the correct setting and (d) there is a residual astigmatic error the axis of which does not coincide with that of the target

on the target that run at 90 degrees to the other three lines (*see Figure 8.12*(c) and (d)). Half of these two lines enter the eye through the right side of the pupil, while the other half enter through the left side. Any vertical displacement of these two lines indicates that the instrument is not along either of the patient's astigmatic axes. The axis of any astigmatism is found by rotating the whole instrument about its anterior–posterior axis until these lines are aligned. The magnitude of the astigmatism is measured by aligning the three lines along both of the astigmatic axes. A complete ray diagram of the Hartinger instrument is given in *Figure 8.13*, and an isometric diagram in *Figure 8.14*.

By inclining the axis of the illuminating system and attaching two small prisms over half of the target's detail, the incident beam is divided into two off-axis beams, each of which contains half of the target's detail. The double slit aperture confines each of these two beams to a small slit region

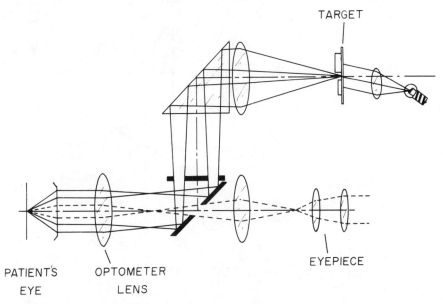

Figure 8.13. Ray diagram of the Hartinger coincidence optometer (Zeiss (Jena))

within the pupil and to either side of its centre (*see Figure 8.14*). Because the double slit aperture of the illuminating system and the circular aperture of the mirror in the viewing system are both imaged in separate regions of the pupillary plane, the viewing system is reflex free.

The amount of light reflected by the retina is only a small percentage of that incident upon it. This means that in order for the target to be clearly seen by the optometrist, its intensity has to be high. In the absence of any other fixation device, this bright stimulus will be a major factor in the control of the patient's accommodation. As the vergence of light from the target varies, so too will the stimulus to accommodation. This means that the technique used to measure the refractive error can effect the results, e.g. if the refractive error is approached from the minus side of the dioptric scale, then accommodation is more likely to be stimulated than if it were approached from the positive side. Generally, this lack of control over the accommodative system results in an increased number of errors.

In order to measure the refractive error in patients with small pupils, it is important to have a small separation between the two beams that enter the patient's eye. Zeiss (Jena) have set this at about 2 mm. The problem with this is that the sensitivity of the optometer is dependent upon this separation: the greater the separation, the greater the amount of displacement per dioptre of error. The designers therefore have to compromise between sensitivity and ability to measure refractive errors in patients with small pupils.

A similar compromise has to be made between target illumination and sensitivity. The more light that is put into the eye, the more light that will

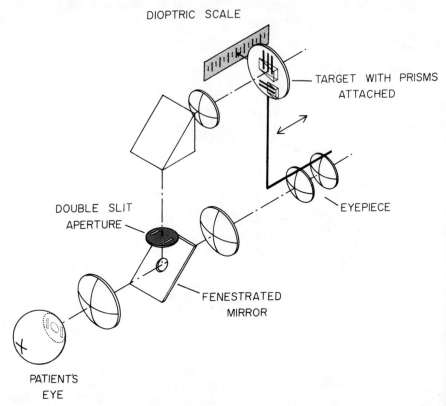

Figure 8.14. Isometric diagram of the Hartinger coincidence optometer (Zeiss (Jena))

be reflected from the retinal layers and the easier it will be to make a setting. However, increasing the illumination also reduces the pupil size and therefore requires an instrument with a smaller separation between the two incident beams, which in turn is less sensitive.

Topcon make a series of three optometers that are optically similar to the Zeiss (Jena) instrument. Two of these, the RM 100 and the RM 200, use infra-red light to illuminate the target rather than visible light. This modification improves the optometer in two ways: first, because the patient can no longer see the target, his accommodative state is unaffected by the vergence of light from it and, second, the pupil size is not affected by the target illumination. The Topcon infra-red optometers incorporate a small television camera and monitor that convert the invisible infra-red radiation returning from the patient's retina into a visible display.

Infra-red optometers

Introduction

A major problem with optometers that use visible light is that they do not have sufficient control over the patient's accommodation. The targets for these instruments have all been visible to the patient. As the vergence of light from the target is altered so too is the stimulus to accommodation.

This problem of patient accommodation can be overcome if the target is made invisible to the patient and if the patient is given a separate fixation target which is specifically designed to encourage a relaxation of accommodation. There are several optometers that have adopted this approach. They have all made the measuring target invisible by placing, in front of the light source, a filter which only transmits the infra-red radiations. They have then either replaced the observer with an electronic focus detector or used some sort of image converter within the viewing system that converts the infra-red radiation reflected by the retina into visible light. This light is then used by the operator to correctly focus the target on the patient's retina. The majority of commercially produced instruments have adopted the former approach as it has the added advantage of being fully objective (i.e. not requiring any judgement to be made by the operator) and therefore operable by personnel with only a limited amount of training.

The chromatic aberration of the human eye means that the estimate of the refractive error with infra-red light will be considerably more hyperopic than it would be if visible light were used. To compensate for this, the manufacturers of infra-red optometers calibrate their instruments with subjective measurements of the refraction. They simply set the dioptric scales of their instruments to give, as near as possible, the same result as subjective measures.

Over the last few years there has been a tremendous increase in the number of infra-red optometers on the market (*see* Guyton, 1980). In the following discussion of these instruments, three of the earlier designs, upon which a good deal of research has been conducted, will be considered. Each of these instruments demonstrates one of the three basic principles upon which all current infra-red optometers are based. These basic principles and the optometers which utilize them are:

1. Grating focus principle: Dioptron Ultima (Coherent Radiation), Auto Ref R–1 (Canon);
2. Retinoscopy: Ophthalmetron (Bausch and Lomb), Auto Refracto-meter NR 1000 (Nikon);
3. Scheiner disc principle: 6600 Auto Refractor (Acuity Systems), $R_x 1$ Auto Refractor (Acuity Systems), Eye-Refractometer RM 200 (Topcon), NIDEK AR-2000 Objective Automatic Refractor (Marco Equipment).

The Dioptron

The Dioptron (*see Figure 8.15*), is a fully objective infra-red refractometer. Once aligned with the eye it will perform a sphere-cylindrical refraction, the results of which are printed out on a small card. The instrument utilizes a technique known as retinal image refraction. This technique is essentially the same as that used in the Rodenstock refractometer, i.e. an image of a mask is formed upon the retina which is viewed by a focus detector (the observer, in the case of the Rodenstock instrument). The vergence of light entering the eye is altered until the detector records that the retinal image of the target is in focus.

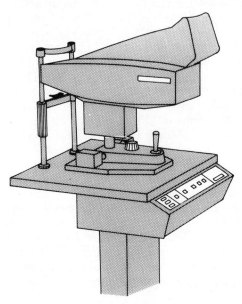

Figure 8.15. The Dioptron (Coherent Radiation)

An isometric diagram of the instrument is shown in *Figure 8.16*. The light source is filtered so as to transmit only the invisible infra-red radiations. This light then passes through a rotating drum in which there are a number of equally spaced slits, the axes of which are parallel to the axis of rotation. The drum acts as a target, an image of which is formed on or near the retina of the patient. Some of the light which makes up this image is reflected back by the retina and is viewed through a mask (composed of bars) by a photocell. The sizes of the gaps in this mask are equal to those of the drum after reflection and refraction through the optics of the instrument and the eye. When the image of the drum is in focus at the plane of this grating and the gaps in the drum are coincident with those of the grating, the amount of light that reaches the photocell is maximum. If the image were to go out of focus or be moved to one side, then the amplitude of the photocell signal would be reduced.

As the drum rotates, its image moves across the grating which produces a fluctuation in the signal from the photocell. The signal reaches a maximum when the gaps coincide and a minimum when the gaps of the drum fall upon the bars of the grating. The maximum alternation of the photocell signal occurs when the image of the drum is in focus upon the grating – i.e. when the image of the drum is sharply focused upon the reflecting plane of the retina.

The amplitude of the photocell signal is internally monitored by the Dioptron as the optometer lens is moved back and forth. The movement of this lens effectively controls the vergence of the light that enters the eye and thus the image plane of the drum. By noting the position of the optometer lens commensurate with maximum photocell alternation an estimation of the patient's refraction is obtained. (The Dioptron actually uses the signal from the photocell to control the position of the lens.)

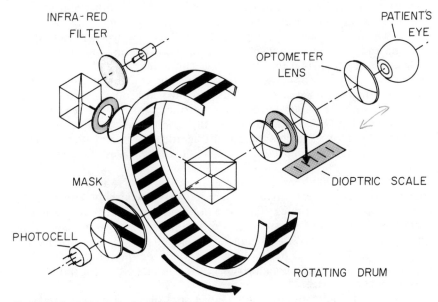

Figure 8.16. An isometric diagram of the Dioptron

After internally recording the refractive state of the patient's eye in one meridian, the Dioptron goes on to measure the refraction in five other meridians. These six measurements are then used to calculate the full refractive state of the patient's eye.

The technique of calculating the full prescription from a series of readings taken along specific meridians has been described by Bennett (1960) and, in theory, only requires measurements along three meridians. However, Long (1974) has pointed out that when the measurements are confined to three meridians, small measurement errors can produce large errors in the computation of the full prescription. Increasing the number of meridians in which a measurement is taken not only increases the confidence with which any prescription is calculated, but also allows the calculation of a 'confidence factor', which indicates to the practitioner the amount of variability encountered in measuring the prescription. If the confidence factor is low then this may indicate that the patient's accommodation fluctuated during the measurement process and would suggest to the practitioner that a repeat measurement may be required.

One of the major problems of refractometers is to keep the accommodation of the patient relaxed during the measurement process. Any acccommodation exerted will result in errors in the measured refractive error. In the Dioptron, accommodation is controlled by the provision of two targets, one for each eye, of a star-burst pattern. The vergence of light from the star-burst pattern to the eye being measured is under the control of the refractometer. It is adjusted during the measurement process so that it will appear fogged by about 1.50 D. It is only after the refractometer has found the most positive measure of the refraction and adjusted the vergence of light from the target to maintain the 1.50 D fog that it performs its final refraction, the results of which are printed out. So as to prevent the eye that is not being measured from influencing the accommodative state, its target, which is the same as that presented to the other eye, is produced out of focus and at a lower intensity to that of the eye being measured.

Because of the strong link between accommodation and convergence, any accommodative effort usually results in some convergence of the eyes. By presenting a binocular target, fusion of which requires zero convergence, Coherent Radiation have added a further control over accommodation. Munnerlyn (1978), who describes the fixation system in detail, states that with the above controls there is no significant tendency to accommodate beyond that experienced with conventional measures of the refractive state.

The Dioptron has been clinically evaluated by Polse and Kerr (1975) who found that its performance compared very favourably with conventional refractive techniques. They did not feel, however, that it could be used as a replacement for subjective refraction because 30 per cent of its findings were in error by more than 0.50 D and 10 per cent by amounts that ranged from 0.75 to 1.62 D. They felt that the major value of this instrument was as a screening instrument or as a subsititute for retinoscopy in optometric practice.

As part of their investigation, Polse and Kerr also evaluated the usefulness of the 'confidence factor' that is provided with each refractive measure. They found that this factor was based upon the astigmatic element of the refraction and hence was of no value in predicting the accuracy of the spherical component. They also found that it was partially dependent upon cylinder axis orientation being generally lower for oblique cylinders than for ones the axes of which were along the principle meridians. They concluded that due to the obvious complexity of this factor and its dependence upon cylinder power and axis, it was of little predictive value to the optometrist.

The Ophthalmetron

The Ophthalmetron refractometer (*see Figure 8.17*), which was made by the Bausch and Lomb Company, utilizes the principle of retinoscopy in order to obtain an estimation of a patient's refraction. The exact mechanism by which it does this is shown in *Figure 8.18*. Light is passed into the patient's eye from the main lamp via an infra-red filter, condenser, chopper drum and two semi-reflecting mirrors. The chopper drum, which rotates so as to intercept the beam of light from the lamp 720 times/second,

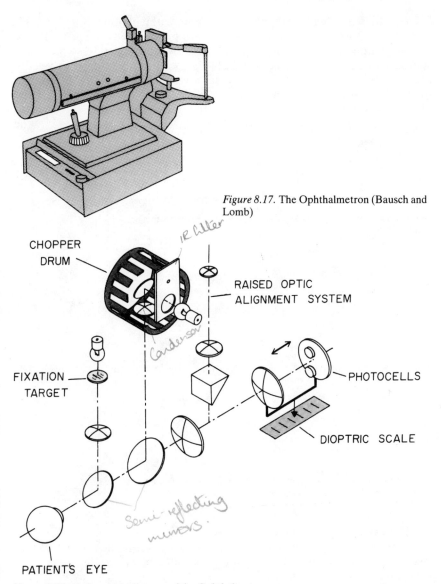

Figure 8.17. The Ophthalmetron (Bausch and Lomb)

CHOPPER DRUM

IR filter

RAISED OPTIC ALIGNMENT SYSTEM

Carderson

FIXATION TARGET

PHOTOCELLS

DIOPTRIC SCALE

Semi-reflecting mirrors.

PATIENT'S EYE

Figure 8.18. An isometric diagram of the Ophthalmetron

produces a moving patch of light upon the retina of the patient. Continuing the analogy between this instrument and retinoscopy, this section of the Ophthalmetron is equivalent to the scanning light source. To view the reflex, Bausch and Lomb have built an electronic observer in the form of a detector lens and a pair of photocells. When the patient's retina is coincident with a point in front of the detector lens, as shown in *Figure 8.19*(a), then a moving patch of light will fall initially on the upper cell and then traverse the photocells. However, when the patient's retina is coincident with a point behind the detector lens, as shown in *Figure*

8.19(b), then a patch of light will again traverse the photocells, only in this case the light will initially fall upon the lower cell. The two photocells are linked to a piece of electronic equipment known as a phase discriminator. This circuit can recognize upon which photocell the light originally fell – i.e. whether there is a 'with' or 'against' movement. The phase discrimina-tor feeds its output to a servo motor which moves the detector lens and photocell assembly until the patient's retina is coincident with the detector lens. In this position, the photocells are simultaneously illuminated by the patch of light.

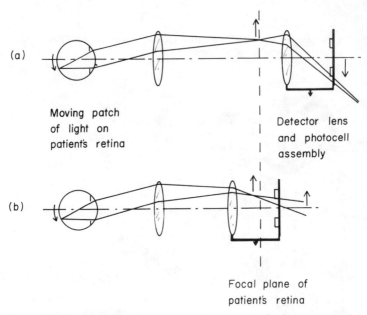

Figure 8.19. The direction of movement at the photocells changes with the position of the detector lens assembly

The position of the detector at this time is a measure of the patient's refractive state along one meridian. In order to measure the refractive state in other meridians and thus obtain a measure of any astigmatism, the instrument is made to gradually rotate around the visual axis while the detector assembly continues to keep the patient's retina coincident with the detector lens.

The position of the detector assembly is plotted out on a piece of graph paper as the instrument rotates. In cases of a spherical refraction, the output will be a straight line, while in cases of astigmatism, the output will be a sine wave where the position of the peaks in the wave represent the axes, and the degree of modulation the amplitude, of the astigmatism (*see Figure 8.20*).

While this type of readout may initially seem a little elaborate in comparison with the digital readouts found in some later instruments, it does allow the operator to assess the reliability of the data. Any variance between the starting and finishing points or any non-sinusoidal changes are usually indicative of unstable accommodation.

In addition to those parts of the Ophthalmetron already discussed, there also exist two other separate optical systems. The first of these is a fixation system for the patient. A target, usually of a distant scene, is viewed through a focusing lens which is positioned so as to slightly fog the target and thus encourage the patient to relax his accommodation. The second optical system is used to align the patient correctly with the instrument. This system is raised, when not in use, so as to be out of the optical path of the detectors. When in use, the infra-red filter normally positioned in front

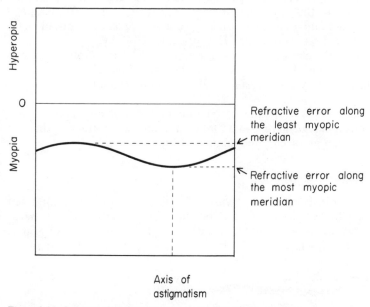

Figure 8.20. Output of the Ophthalmetron from a patient who has compound myopic astigmatism

of the main lamp is replaced by a special stop, an image of which is viewed by the operator after reflection from the patient's cornea. To effect alignment, the instrument is adjusted until this image is aligned with the optics of the instrument.

Two independent reviews of the Ophthalmetron have been published in the literature, the first by Floyd and Garcia (1974) and the second by Bizzell *et al.* (1974). These researchers conducted similar experiments in that they compared the findings of the Ophthalmetron with those of retinoscopy and subjective tests. To avoid any experimenter bias, Bizzell *et al.* (1974) used different experimenters for each of the tests and did not allow any of the experimenters to see any results until all measurements had been completed. The conclusions of the two groups of experimenters were:

1. That the mean spherical response of the three measures of refraction were practically identical;

2. That the variability between the Ophthalmetron and subjective finding was greater than that between retinoscopy and subjective tests. Bizzell's results showed that for spheres, 79.7 per cent of retinoscopies were within 0.50 D of the subjective finding, while only 56.2 per cent of the Ophthalmetron's were. For cylinder powers, 87.4 per cent of retinoscopies were within 0.50 D of the subjective finding, while only 71.5 per cent of the Opthalmetron's were;

3. That the Ophthalmetron tended to give slightly higher cylinder powers than either retinoscopy or subjective tests;

4. That more difficulty was found in obtaining a measurement of the refraction in uncooperative patients with the Ophthalmetron than with retinoscopy or the subjective procedures; Bizzell *et al.* (1974) failed to get an adequate reading in 26 per cent of the people tested. The majority of these were under 12 years old;

5. That the time taken to perform a refraction with the Ophthalmetron was greater than that of retinoscopy when the time taken to align the patient and analyze the results was taken into account.

Bizzell *et al.* (1974) conclude by stating that the main value of the Ophthalmetron may be in research for the monitoring of refractive changes and in the screening of large population groups.

The 6600 Auto-Refractor

The 6600 Auto-Refractor (*see Figure 8.21*) is a fully objective infra-red optometer. Once aligned with the patient's eye it performs a spherocylindrical refraction without the aid of the optometrist. Optically, it is based upon the principles of the Scheiner disc (*see* p.152). Rather than use

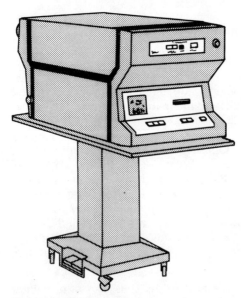

Figure 8.21. The 6600 Auto-Refractor (Acuity Systems)

two pin holes, as in the original Scheiner disc, the 6600 Auto-Refractor uses two light sources both of which are slightly displaced from the optical axis of the illuminating system (*see Figure 8.22*). These sources are both imaged in the plane of the patient's pupil.

The target of the Auto-Refractor is a movable diaphragm. When this diaphragm is not coincident with the reflecting plane of the patient's retina,

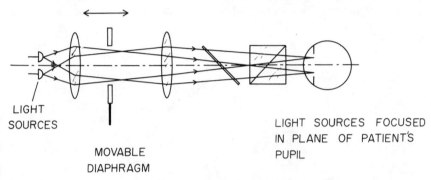

LIGHT
SOURCES

MOVABLE
DIAPHRAGM

LIGHT SOURCES FOCUSED
IN PLANE OF PATIENT'S
PUPIL

Figure 8.22. The light sources of the 6600 Auto-Refractor are imaged in the plane of the patient's pupil

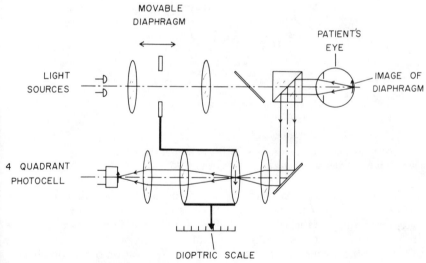

MOVABLE
DIAPHRAGM

PATIENT'S
EYE

LIGHT
SOURCES

IMAGE OF
DIAPHRAGM

4 QUADRANT
PHOTOCELL

DIOPTRIC SCALE

Figure 8.23. The diaphragms image upon the retina of the patient is viewed by the four quadrant photocell

two blurred images of it will be produced at the retina, one from each of the two light sources. A measure of the patient's refraction is obtained by moving the diaphragm back and forth until these two images are superimposed.

In operation, the two light sources are alternately flashed. If the diaphragm is sharply focused upon the retina, then no apparent movement will be detected because the two images are superimposed. The four quadrant photocell situated in the measuring system is designed to detect any movement (*see Figure 8.23*). The rather elaborate system of lenses in the path of the photocell is necessary to remove the corneal reflex.

In order to detect and measure any astigmatism, the Auto-Refractor has two additional light sources which are aligned perpendicularly to the first two such that all four are equally spaced on the circumference of a circle (*see Figure 8.24*). The second pair of light sources are alternately turned on at a different frequency to that of the first pair. If the axis of the second

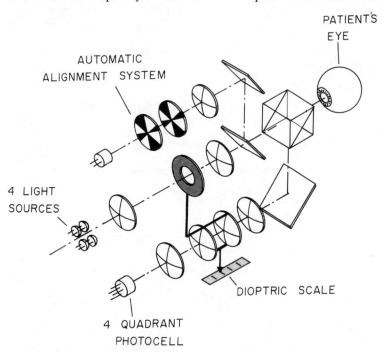

Figure 8.24. An isometric diagram of the 6600 Auto-Refractometer showing the alignment system, the illuminating system and the viewing system

pair does not coincide with the axis of astigmatism, then the axis of the images falling upon the detector will not coincide with its own axis. The detector recognizes this situation and rotates itself and the sources until the image motion coincides with the detector axis. This position is recorded as the axis of the patient's astigmatism. When the position of the diaphragm gives a detector null for the first pair of sources, it is recorded as the sphere power. The degree of movement, seen at the detector as the second pair of light sources is alternated, is then converted into a measure of the magnitude of the astigmatism.

Transverse alignment of the instrument is obtained by the operator who views the corneal reflex produced by the four light sources. Axial alignment is obtained automatically by a separate optical system which also utilizes the corneal reflex. This latter system ensures that the light sources are focused in the plane of the patient's pupil. During the measurement process, the eye being measured views a dull green fixation light through a plus lens and pin hole aperture. This type of fixation light is claimed to decrease the stimuli for accommodation.

A clinical evaluation of the instrument has been conducted by Hill (1973) who found that 81 per cent of spherical findings and 92 per cent of the cylindrical components were within ±0.50 D of their subjective findings. However, only 86 per cent of the cylindrical axes were found to be within ±10 degrees. Unfortunately, Hill does not break down the cylindrical axis data into groups of varying cylinder power and, hence, it is impossible to say whether or not this inaccuracy is simply the result of large errors in the measurement of low-power cylinders.

In a later evaluation by Pappas, Anderson and Briese (1978), only 56 per cent of the readings from normal patients were found to be within ±0.50 D of their subjective findings, 21 per cent having an error greater than ±1.00 D. In analyzing the accuracy of the Auto-Refractor at determining cylinder axis, Pappas and his colleagues removed the data from those patients with less than 0.50 D of astigmatism. They found that 82 per cent of the remaining patients' axis errors were within ±10 degrees and 54 per cent within ±5 degrees of their subjective findings.

Pappas, Anderson and Briese (1978) also measured the refractive error of a number of pathological eyes with the Auto-Refractor and found the results to be worse than those for normal eyes. They concluded that the instrument is not sufficiently accurate to allow its results to be prescribed and that it is most reliable in those cases where the media is clear and where retinoscopy can be quickly and easily performed.

Recently developed subjective instruments

American Optical SR III subjective refraction system

The SR III refractor (*see Figure 8.25*) is a box-shaped instrument that contains a series of test targets and a variable-power lens system based

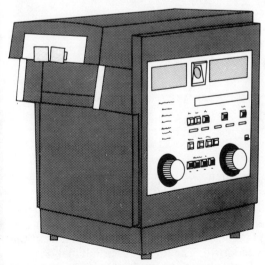

Figure 8.25. American Optical SR III subjective refractometer

upon a design first produced by Guyton (1972). In operation, the patient is required to adjust the power of the lens system in accordance with the instructions given by the operator. Following a sequence of such adjustments, the patient's refractive error is displayed on the side of the instrument.

Optics

The optics of the SR III can be viewed as a development upon the simple optometer discussed earlier. The patient views an aerial image of a target through an optometer lens rather than the target itself. This is advantageous because the aerial image can be made to have an astigmatic

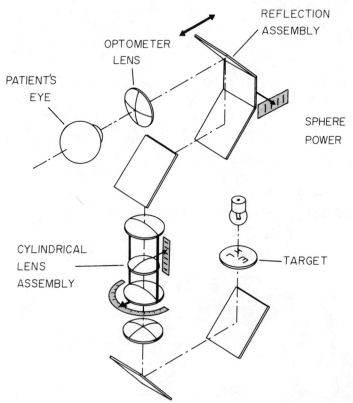

Figure 8.26. An isometric diagram of the optics of the SR III subjective refractometer

component that can then be used to measure any astigmatism in the patient.

A simplified diagram of the optical system of the SR III is given in *Figure 8.26*. Sphere power is adjusted by moving the reflector assembly back and forth, while cylindrical power is adjusted by moving the central lens of the cylindrical lens assembly back and forth. The three lenses that make up the cylindrical lens assembly are all astigmatic. The central lens has its axis at

90 degrees to the other two lenses and has a power equal to the combined equivalent power of the other two lenses. The axis of any cylindrical component is varied by rotating the cylindrical lens assembly around the optical axis.

Target design

If an astigmatic patient views a point light source placed at the far point of his astigmatic meridians, then the point will appear as a short line the axis of which corresponds to one of the axes of the astigmatism. If the same patient were to view a line of point sources, then each point would be seen as a short line (*see Figure 8.27(b)*). The axis of astigmatism, in this situation, can be found by asking the patient to rotate the line of point

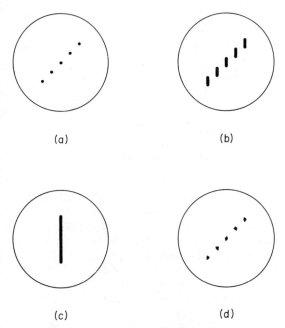

(a)   (b)

(c)   (d)

Figure 8.27. (a) Target composed of a line of dots;
(b) appearance of the target to a patient who has astigmatism, the axis of which does not coincide with that of the dots;
(c) appearance of the target when the axis of the patient's astigmatism coincides with that of the dots; (d) appearance of the target in a case of low-power astigmatism

sources until the short lines appear aligned (*see Figure 8.27(c)*). The problem with this type of target is that it is insensitive to small astigmatic errors. When a patient with a small astigmatic error views this type of target, each point of light is seen as an indistinct line similar to that shown in *Figure 8.27*(d). The sensitivity of this type of target can, however, be improved by placing a cylindrical lens in front of the line of points with the

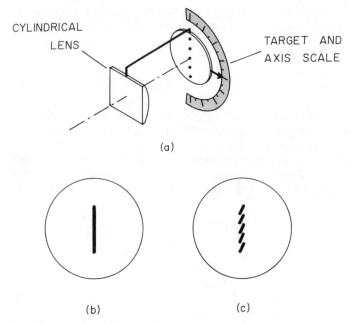

CYLINDRICAL
LENS

TARGET AND
AXIS SCALE

(a)

(b)   (c)

Figure 8.28. (a) The cylindrical lens is attached to the dot type target;
(b) the appearance of the dot target to a non astigmatic patient
through the cylindrical lens; (c) appearance of the target to an
astigmatic patient whose axis does not coincide with that of the target

lens axis at 90 degrees to the line (*see Figure 8.28*(a)). This cylinder will
make each point appear as a line which, for the non astigmatic patient, will
lie along the line of points (*see Figure 8.28*(b)). When a patient with
astigmatism views this target, the ocular astigmatism will combine with the
astigmatism of the lens. If the axes of the two do not coincide, then the
resultant cylinder will be at an axis different to that of the line of point
sources and the patient will see a jagged line (*see Figure 8.28*(c)). The axis
of astigmatism can, in this situation, be measured by rotating the target and
lens until the jaggedness in the line has been removed.

The sequence of measurements with the SR III

1. The patient is presented with a target composed of a line of points seen
    through the astigmatic lens. The sphere power is adjusted until the
    patient sees either a clear jagged line (some astigmatism present at an
    axis other than that of the line of points) or a clear straight line (no
    astigmatism, or astigmatism along the axis of the line of points).
2. The line of points is rotated until any jaggedness has been removed.
    The sphere is then adjusted until the line is perfectly clear.
3. The patient is presented with a cross of points with axes at 45 degrees
    to the setting made with the single line of points. The patient is
    instructed to adjust the cylindrical component until any jaggedness has
    been removed.

4. The visual acuity of the patient is reduced with a plus sphere, the power of which is then gradually reduced until maximum acuity is obtained.

Advantages of the SR III over objective optometers

1. Because the SR III uses cylindrical lenses to measure the astigmatism a fluctuation in accommodation during the measurement process will not affect the measured astigmatic error. All the previously described objective optometers, with the exception of the 6600, measure astigmatism by taking a series of readings along different meridians. Any fluctuation of accommodation during this process will alter the computed astigmatic error.
2. The final presciptions can be prescribed.
3. At the end of the measurement cycle, the patient views a high contrast letter chart which is fogged by a +2.00 DS (dioptre spheres). The power of this sphere is then gradually reduced to give the maximum visual acuity. This technique (which is almost identical to the sphere check carried out by optometrists during a conventional refractor examination) will give, with time, what has been shown to be an excellent measurement of the spherical component.
4. The visual acuity of the patient is recorded.

Residual problems of the SR III as a means of routine refraction

1. The instrument refracts monocularly and contains no facilities for binocularly balancing the final prescription.
2. The method of adjusting the cylindrical and spherical components, i.e. until the jaggedness has been removed, does not always have a clear end point due to the aberrations of the eye. This point is demonstrated in *Figure 8.29* where it can be seen that the edges of the short lines seen by the eye pass through the periphery of the pupil while the centre of the short lines passes through the centre of the pupil. If the refractive

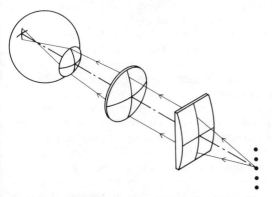

Figure 8.29. The edges of the short lines produced by the cylindrical lens are seen through the edge of the pupil while the centre is seen through the pupil's centre

error measured through the different regions of the pupil is not the same then the short lines will not appear straight, but will be curved at their ends. Any curvature will make the setting of the instrument to a position where the jaggedness has been removed difficult as there will always be some residual jaggedness.

3.   The SR III uses a psychophysical test known as 'continuous adjustment' which means that the patient is allowed to alter the vergence of the light that enters the eye along a continuous scale until the short lines appear aligned. A far better psychophysical technique, better in that it is easier for the patient and thus gives a better estimate of the error, is that known as 'forced choice'. With this technique, the patient would be shown two views of, in this case, a jagged line and asked which was the better of the two. An example of a forced choice technique that is regularly used in optometric practice is the crossed cylinder test. This test has been shown, with time, to be extremely reliable and accurate in the measurement of astigmatism.

Woo and Woodruff (1978) conducted a clinical trial of the SR III refraction system in which the results from a secretary, trained in the use of the SR III, were compared with the results obtained by final year students and staff of the university using conventional subjective techniques. They concluded from a study of 580 eyes that the two techniques gave practically identical results. Most of the differences were within the tolerances for different examiners and/or different methods as calculated by other researchers.

American Optical SR IV subjective refraction system

Several of the problems relating to the SR III refractor have been overcome by American Optical with the development of a new subjective refractor, the SR IV. Optically, this instrument is based upon the same principles as the SR III. The jagged line targets have, however, been replaced with a cross cylinder system (Simulcross). This system simultaneously presents the patient with two targets, one viewed through each of the flipped positions of a crossed cylinder. The patient reports which of the two looks clearer, and the operator responds by pressing the appropriate button. The power or axis of the cylinder is then automatically changed by a given amount and the patient is asked again which of the two is clearer. The amount by which the cylinder is changed is dependent upon the power of the cylinder already within the system. If, for example, the SR IV optics contain the equivalent of an 0.25 DC correction, then the step changes in axis will be fairly large. If, on the other hand, the optics contain the equivalent of 2.00 DC, then the axis changes would be much smaller.

American Optical now also manufacture a data printer for the SR IV. Its printout gives details of unaided and final acuities as well as the final prescription and can, by feeding in the old prescription to the SR IV, be used to calculate the over refraction as well as the new refraction.

The Humphrey Vision Analyzer (Humphrey Instruments)

The Humphrey Vision Analyzer (*see Figure 8.30*) is a remote subjective refractor. It differs from the American Optical SR III in that it was designed to be used by an optometrist and it enables a full binocular refraction to be performed, including tests of phoria, fixation disparity,

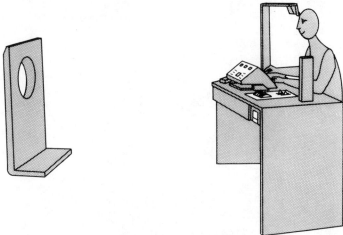

Figure 8.30. The Humphrey Vision Analyzer

stereopsis and reading addition. It contains three novel features which differentiate it from all other subjective refractors.

1. It utilizes a new type of variable-power lens which was originally developed by Alvarez (*see* Alvarez, 1978, for a description).
2. It removes all instrumentation, such as refracting units and trial frames, from the immediate vicinity of the patient's face.
3. It utilizes a completely new method for the measurement of astigmatic errors.

Alvarez variable-power lenses

Each Alvarez variable-power lens is composed of two elements that can be moved with respect to each other along two mutually perpendicular axes. When the two lenses are in exact register with each other, the overall power of the lens combination is zero. This can be seen more easily from an examination of *Figure 8.31*. In this figure each of the elements has been divided into small sections and the average spherical and astigmatic power of each section has been marked. It is important to remember that the elements themselves are *not* divided into sections, but are continuously variable across their surfaces. This division has been made solely to aid in the description of how these lenses function. It can be seen from *Figure 8.31* that, when in exact register, each section within each element is exactly neutralized by the similarly positioned section of the other element – i.e. the combined power of both elements is zero across the entire surface of the lens.

If one of the elements were to be moved along the <u>horizontal</u> axis by one section, then for every overlapping section the total power of the two elements is +1.00 DS. Continued movement along this axis will further increase this <u>spherical power</u>. Movement of this element in the opposite direction will create negative power over all the overlapping sections. Thus, by moving one element along the horizontal axis, we have created a variable-power spherical lens.

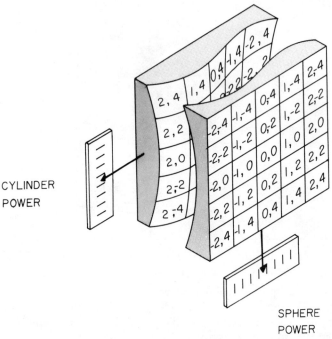

CYLINDER
POWER

SPHERE
POWER

Figure 8.31. Schematic diagram of the Alvarez lens. The first number within each cell represents the average spherical power of that part of the lens while the second number represents the cylindrical power

It can also be seen from *Figure 8.31* that if the other element is moved along the vertical axis then the spherical powers remain constant while the astigmatic powers vary. Again, the amount of variation in astigmatic power is constant over all the remaining overlapping sections. Movement of both elements produces a combined spherico-cylindrical power.

In summary, a single Alvarez lens, which is composed of two elements, is capable of producing a sphere–cylinder combination by moving one of its elements along a horizontal axis and its other element along a vertical axis. The axis of the cylindrical component remains constant and need not coincide with either the vertical or horizontal meridians.

Removal of instrumentation from immediate vicinity of the patient's face

The Humphrey Vision Analyzer does not require any lenses to be placed immediately in front of the patient's face. The patient is simply positioned, with the patient's head resting gently against a support, and told to look into a large, concave mirror placed some 3 m in front of the eyes. Within this mirror, the patient sees targets, such as Snellen letters, the vergence of light from which can be varied in order to effect a refraction.

The basis of this technique, which Humphrey calls 'remote refraction', is shown in *Figure 8.32*. In this figure, the Alvarez variable-power unit has zero power and the target is brought to focus by the condenser at the focal plane of the mirror. The image of the target is therefore seen, after

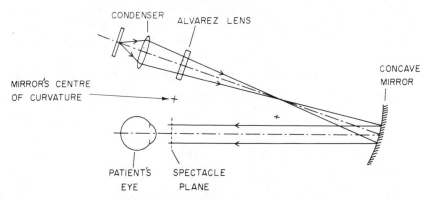

Figure 8.32. The optical arrangement of the lens unit in the Humphrey Vision Analyzer, the concave mirror and the patient's spectacle plane. After Bennett (1977)

reflection by the mirror, at infinity. When the power of the Alvarez lens is changed, the vergence of light that enters the eye from the target is also changed. Because the lens unit, the spectacle plane and the centre of curvature of the mirror all lie in the same plane, it can be shown that any change in the power of the lens unit results in an equal change in the vergence of light at the spectacle plane. In other words, it is as if the lens unit were placed in the spectacle plane.

Method of measuring astigmatic errors

A cylinder of any desired power and axis can be obtained by the combination of two cylinders the axes of which are fixed, but the powers of which are variable. This is the basis upon which the Humphrey Vision Analyzer works. Rather than have a rotatable variable astigmatic lens, it has two variable astigmatic units at fixed axes, one with its axes at 180 and 90 degrees, the other with its axes at 45 and 135 degrees.

The utilization of astigmatic units at fixed axes lends itself to a completely new way of establishing refractive errors. By considering an astigmatic error as being composed of two components at 45 degrees to each other, it can be shown that when one of the components has been found and placed in the refractor, the remaining cylindrical error will be along the axis of the other component. The relevance of this becomes obvious when we consider the design of the targets used for the assessment of astigmatism and the recommended refractive technique.

The Humphrey Vision Analyzer measures each component individually by presenting the patient with a series of three lines oriented along the power axis of the component not being measured (*see Figure 8.33*). When the correct power of the component being measured has been found, the residual blur will be along the axis of the target's central line, i.e. this line will appear clear except at its ends.

The task of finding each of the astigmatic components has therefore been reduced to that of adjusting the power of the 45/135 unit until a set of vertical lines appears clear and then adjusting the power of the 90/180 degree unit until a set of 45 degree lines appears clear. The sensitivity of this setting can be improved with the use of a bias cylinder the axis of which coincides with that of the target's central line. This bias cylinder, in cases of

Bias cylinder axis and power axis
of the component not being measured

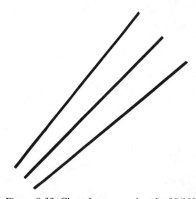

Figure 8.33. Chart for measuring the 90/180 component of any astigmatism

low astigmatism, makes the central line appear very much darker than the other two lines. The patient is instructed to alter the power of the appropriate astigmatic unit until the two outer lines are equally blurred, a setting which can be made with great precision. In the Humphrey Vision Analyzer the bias cylinder has a power of 4.00 D. A small computer built into the Vision Analyzer records the positions of the lens elements and computes the combined cylindrical power and axis. The results are provided in digital format on the console of the instrument.

For near-vision testing, a pair of prisms is placed in front of the patient's eye. These allow the patient to converge and depress the eyes while viewing targets presented by the same system as that used for distance testing. While this is identical, optically, to the situation experienced by a patient viewing a near hand-held target, perceptually it is not. Because perceived distance influences the near response, the accommodation and convergence exerted by the patient with the Humphrey Vision Analyzer may not equal that used in the normal environment.

Kratz and Flom (1977) have measured the reliability and validity of refractive error measurements with the Humphrey Vision Analyzer. They compared the results obtained by a technician, who had 150 h experience with the Analyzer, with those of an experienced optometrist using a refractor head. Their results show that the differences between the two refractive techniques were no greater than the differences obtained between two successive measures taken either with the refractor head or the Humphrey Vision Analyzer. They concluded that the results obtained with the Humphrey Vision Analyzer, using the method of measuring astigmatism just outlined, were as reliable and valid as those obtained with the conventional refractor head and the Jackson cross cylinder.

Elmstrom (1977) has discussed some of the patient management problems encountered with the Humphrey Vision Analyzer. One of the major ones is that of monitoring the patient's head position. The light that enters each of the patient's eyes is confined to a beam the diameter of which is approximately 20 mm at the eye. If the patient moves to one side, then his eyes may no longer fall within the beam with the result that the patient will no longer see the target. When this occurs, the patient has to be realigned by the optometrist before the test can continue.

A shortcoming of the Humphrey Vision Analyzer is that the optometrist cannot perform a retinoscopic examination or any other type of objective refraction while the patient is seated at the Analyzer. Having to rely totally upon subjective procedures can, in certain cases, lengthen the examination time and over-fatigue the patient. To overcome this problem, Humphrey Instruments recommend that optometrists refract over the patient's previous prescription. This greatly reduces the refraction time and, because the in-built computer has the facility of automatically compounding the power of the patient's spectacles with the over refraction findings, it does not result in any tedious calculations.

The Humphrey Vision Analyzer as a whole is doubtlessly one of the most important developments in the field of refraction that has occurred since the development of the refractor head. At present, its high cost and sophistication are likely to deter many optometrists from incorporating this instrument into their consulting rooms. Its innovative ideas will, however, certainly shape the development of future optometric instrumentation.

References

ALVAREZ, L. W. (1978). Development of variable-focus lenses and a new refractor. *Journal of the American Optometric Association*, **49**, 24

BENNETT, A. G. (1960). Refraction by automation. *Optician*, **139**, 5

BENNETT, A. G. (1977). Some novel optical features of the Humphrey Vision Analyzer. *Optician*, **173**, 7

BIZZELL, J. W., HENDRICKS, J. C., GOLDBERG, M. F., PATEL, M. K. and ROBBINS, G. F. (1974). Clinical evaluation of an infrared refracting instrument. *Archives of Ophthalmology*, **92**, 103

BRADFORD, R. T. and LAWSON, L. J. (1954). Clinical evaluation of the Rodenstock refractometer. *Archives of Opthalmology*, **51**, 695

CHARMAN, W. N. and JENNINGS, J. A. M. (1976). Objective measurements of the longitudinal chromatic aberration of the human eye. *Vision Research*, **16**, 999

ELMSTROM, G. (1977). Management consideration of the Humphrey Vision Analyzer. *Journal of the American Optometric Association*, **48**, 1293

FLOYD, R. P. and GARCIA, G. (1974). The Ophthalmetron. *Archives of Ophthalmology*, **92**, 10

GUYTON, D. (1972). *Cylindrical Lens Systems for Simultaneous Bimeridonal Measurements in a Lens Measuring Instrument.* US patent 3 664 631

GUYTON, D. L. (1980). Automated clinical refraction. In *Refraction and Clinical Optics,* Ch. 67, p. 1. Edited by A. Safir. Harper and Row, Hagerstown

HILL, J. F. (1973). Comparison of computerised refraction with standard refractive technique. *Optometric Weekly,* **64,** 1279

HOBBS, F. I. and SCHIMEK, R. A. (1956). The clinical value of the Rodenstock refractometer. *American Journal of Ophthalmology,* **42,** 59

KRATZ, L. D. and FLOM, M. C. (1977). The Humphrey Vision Analyzer: Reliability and validity of refractive error measures. *American Journal of Optometry and Physiological Optics,* **54,** 653

LONG, W. F. (1974). A mathematical analysis of multi-meridonal refractometry. *American Journal of Optometry and Physiological Optics,* **51,** 260

MILLODOT, M. and O'LEARY, D. (1978). The discrepancy between retinoscopic and subjective measurements: Effects of age. *American Journal of Optometry and Physiological Optics,* **55,** 309

MUNNERLYN, C. R. (1978). An optical system for an automatic eye refractor. *Optical Engineering,* **17,** 627

O'LEARY, D. and MILLODOT, M. (1978). The discrepancy between retinoscopic and subjective refraction: Effect of light polarisation. *American Journal of Optometry and Physiological Optics,* **55,** 553

PAPPAS, C. J., ANDERSON, D. R. and BRIESE, F. W. (1978). Clinical evaluation of the 6600 Autorefractor. *Archives of Ophthalmology,* **96,** 993

POLSE, K. A. and KERR, M. E. (1975). An objective optometer. *Archives of Ophthalmology,* **93,** 225

VOLK, D. (1955). Objective methods of refraction. *American Journal of Ophthalmology,* **39,** 719

WOO, G. C. and WOODRUFF, M. E. (1978). The AO SR III subjective refraction system: Comparison with phoropter measures. *American Journal of Optometry and Physiological Optics,* **55,** 591

9

Trial case lenses and refracting units

Introduction

In performing a refraction the majority of practitioners utilize a set of spherical and cylindrical lenses of known power. These lenses are called trial lenses. Trial lenses may be individually mounted such that they can be placed in a special spectacle frame, known as a trial frame, or they may be mounted in a refracting unit. When individually mounted, they are normally sold in sets contained within either a wooden or plastic case. For this reason, these lenses are normally referred to as trial case lenses or trial sets.

Before the types of trial sets available and the advantages and disadvantages of refracting units are described, additive lens systems and the problems of near vision effectivity will be discussed. With an understanding of these topics, the reader should be able to see how errors may occur between what the optometrist measures in his consulting room and what is finally dispensed to the patient.

Additive lens systems

When more than one lens is placed within a trial frame or refracting unit, the back-vertex power of the combination is taken as the algebraic sum of the individual lens powers. Unfortunately, the true, or effective, power of the combination is often different to the algebraic sum. The magnitude of the discrepancy is dependent upon the power, thickness, form and position of the lenses used. Generally, the discrepancy is small on lenses the combined powers of which are below 4 D.

The discrepancy between the true back-vertex power and the algebraic sum of the individual lenses' back-vertex powers was noted back in 1912 when von Rohr first introduced the back-vertex system as a means of classifying trial lenses. The first person to effect a solution to the problem was Kellner (1918). Kellner stated that the back-vertex power of a combination of any two lenses will equal the algebraic sum of their individual powers when the following criterion are satisfied:

1. All the lenses are either planoconvex or planoconcave and when used in combination with each other have their plane surfaces facing each other;
2. All the lenses have the same centre thickness;
3. The separation of the two lenses is kept constant.

In addition, Kellner stated that the cylindrical lens (if any) should be placed in the front cell of the trial frame and that, should there be no spherical error, a glass plate must be placed in the rear cell the thickness of which is the same as the centre thickness of the spherical lenses.

In 1915, Bausch and Lomb started to make trail cases (known as the precision trial case) and trial frames based upon the Kellner principle. The limitation of constant centre thickness meant that the overall diameter of the lenses had to be kept small. The precision trial-case lenses had a diameter of only 15 mm.

In 1923, another patent on additive vertex-power trial lenses was issued to Tillyer (1923). Tillyer's principle stated that the front surface of the ocular lens need not be plane, as in Kellner's system, but could adopt any curvature provided that it was held constant for all the trial lenses and provided that the centre thickness of the spherical lenses was kept constant. It should be noted that Kellner's principle is essentially a special case of Tillyer's principle.

Tillyer stated that the principle he proved for two lenses could be applied to a combination of any number of lenses. Consequently, a number of 'additive' refracting units were manufactured which were based solely upon the Tillyer principle. Unfortunately, Tillyer was wrong. Lang and Marg (1975) have shown that, while Tillyer's principle is correct for stacks of two lenses, there is no simple additive system that can predict the absolute value of the back-vertex power for stacks of more than two lenses.

Near-vision effectivity

The back-vertex power of a lens system is measured with parallel light incident on the front surface. However, the effective power of a lens system does not necessarily equal the back-vertex power when the incident light is other than parallel. The discrepancy between the effective power and back-vertex power is dependent upon centre thickness and only becomes significant on plus lenses of moderate and high power. Bennett (1966) describes a series of lens combinations all with the same back-vertex power (+16.00 D), but with near-vision effectivities that vary over a range of 0.50 D. Bennett (1966) points out that the ideal situation for a trial case or refracting unit is where the near-vision effectivity of the test lenses closely approximates that of the prescribed lens. Unfortunately, the additive lens systems of Kellner and Tillyer have near-vision effectivities which differ markedly from that of prescription lenses.

While this problem was realized by Mayer back in 1920, very little was done about it until 1956 when a British Ministry of Health committee produced a report on trial lens forms (British Standard, 1959). The committee concluded that no single form of lens was ideal from all standpoints, but they suggested that the additive principles of the Kellner system should be retained in a trial case with the modification that the cylindrical lens should now be placed in the rear cell of the trial frame. They claimed that by doing this:

1. The effective cylinder power remained constant for both distance and near;
2. Spherical lenses no longer need to be of constant thickness and therefore larger apertures could be used;
3. When testing near vision, the combination more closely resembled that of prescription lenses and thus any difference between back-vertex power and effective power at near was likely to be similar in the trial lenses and spectacle lenses.

The proposals of the British Ministry of Health were later incorporated in the British Standard 3162 *Ophthalmic Trial Case Lenses* (1959). While this standard does not specify that lenses must follow the modified Kellner principle, as mentioned above, it does lay down rules and regulations regarding the tolerances on lenses in trial cases.

Trial case lenses

Currently produced trial case lenses fall into three main groups, namely full aperture lenses, reduced aperture lenses and additive vertex sets.

Full aperture lenses

Full aperture lenses are approximately 38 mm in diameter and are made in a biconcave or biconvex form. They do not conform to any of the additive lens principles previously mentioned, but are preferred by many practitioners because they do not obscure the patient's face.

Reduced aperture lenses

Reduced aperture lenses are approximately 20 mm in diameter and are supported in a mount the diameter of which is 38 mm. They are of planoconcave or planoconvex* form and have been designed with the intention that the curved surface should face the eye. Failure to do this can, on high-power plus lenses, result in significant errors between the marked power and the back-vertex power. Bennett (1966) calculates that the error would be about 0.25 D on a +12.00 D lens. The power marked on the trial lens is the power of curved surface and not the back-vertex power, as is assumed by most practitioners. The designers of these lenses intended

* Rodenstock make a reduced aperture set in which the lenses are produced in a curved form.

them to be used for both neutralization and refraction. For neutralization, the curved surface of the trial lenses should be placed against the curved surface of the spectacle lens. Bennett (1966) feels that the design of trial lenses should no longer be influenced by a requirement for neutralization. It should be assumed that spectacle lenses are checked with a focimeter.

Additive vertex sets

Additive vertex sets, which have an aperture of about 20 mm, have been designed to comply with the recommendations of the British Ministry of Health committee. The cylindrical lenses of these sets should be placed in the rear cell of the trial frame. The obvious difficulty of being able to record the cylinder axis when a sphere lens is in place is overcome by using transparent mounts for the sphere lenses.

Phoropters

Refracting units, or phoropters, are designed to provide the optometrist with a convenient way of placing trial lenses in front of the patient's eyes during a refraction. The word phoropter stems from two words: phoro, meaning muscle testing, and optometer, meaning refraction. The word phoropter is still accurate today as most phoropters, or refracting units, contain both sets of prisms for the testing of 'phorias' and lenses for performing a refraction.

The first phoropter, that in any way resembled today's phoropters, was developed by De Zeng in 1908. De Zeng's phoropter consisted of a series of four discs, each having a maximum of eight lenses glazed in apertures situated around the edge. By rotating the discs, lens powers from +15.00 to −20.00 D could be obtained at the sight holes of the instrument. Later on two additional smaller discs were added that contained cylindrical lenses. To obtain the correct axis for the cylinders, the discs were rotated about the sight hole.

Most modern refracting units contain the sphere and cylindrical lenses on three discs. The wheel closest to the patient's eye usually contains the high-power spheres, the second disc contains the low-power spheres and the third disc contains the cylindrical lenses. The two sphere wheels are normally connected via a gearing arrangement that enables the sphere power to be incremented or decremented by a single knob, in 0.25 D steps, across the whole range of the instrument. In modern refracting units, the cylindrical axis setting is made by a single knob and thereafter the cylindrical lenses fall into place, through a system of planetary gears, at the same axis setting. This arrangement speeds up the normal refractive procedures as the optometrist does not have to set the axis of the cylinder every time he changes the cylindrical lens power.

In addition to the discs that contain the spheres and cylinders, most refracting units include at least one other disc which contains an assortment of lenses such as occluders, Maddox rods, +1.50 D lens for retinoscopy, pin holes, polaroids and dissociating prisms. Attached to the front of most refracting units, on arms that allow them to be swung in front of the sight hole, are sets of Risley prisms and cross cylinders. On some of the later units, the axes of the cross cylinders are linked to the axis setting knob of the cylindrical lenses so that, when checking the axis of a cylinder, rotation of the cylindrical lens automatically produces a rotation of the cross cylinder.

Advantages of refracting units

The main advantage of refracting units is that they speed up the refraction process. Other advantages are:

1. They are more comfortable for patients. The design and weight of a trial frame with lenses in place is such that they are invariably exceedingly uncomfortable when worn for more than a few minutes;
2. The lenses do not become so greased. On some refracting units the lenses are actually protected by small, removable cover slips which are placed over the sight holes;
3. The axis of any cylindrical correction can be read off from the refractor head with greater accuracy. This is particularly so when optometrists use drop cell trial frames, in which the lens can wobble around a lot, and when the cylindrical correction requires more than one cylindrical lens to be placed in the trial frame;
4. Additivity errors can be reduced. Because the lenses within a refracting unit will always occupy the same position, it is possible to design the unit so that additivity errors are small (*see* pp. 185–186). Two refracting units, the American Optical Ultramatic and the Topcon Vision Tester, claim to have additive lens systems incorporated. As it is impossible to design an additive system for more than two lenses, it must be assumed that these manufacturers have simply designed their units to keep additivity errors low.

Disadvantages of refracting units

The main disadvantages are:

1. It is not possible to check the back-vertex power of a lens combination with the focimeter. Optometrists, therefore, have to rely upon the integrity of the manufacturer when they prescribe from these units. Marg (1980) has reported several instances where lenses within a refractor are either of incorrect power or are mounted back to front;
2. Refracting units hide the patient's face;
3. It is difficult, if not impossible, to do a cover test through a refracting unit;
4. If the patient tilts his head slightly during a refraction, then any cylindrical correction will be prescribed off axis;
5. Because the cylindrical lenses are in front of the spheres, their effective power at near will be different to that of the prescribed lenses (*see* Near-vision effectivity, pp. 186–187).

Summary

Refracting units offer the optometrist advantages in both speed and convenience of use. In the majority of cases, errors due to non additivity of lens powers and errors due to different effectivity between refractor head and spectacle prescription are so small that they need not be considered by the optometrist. However, in cases where the refractive error is high, particularly high plus, a more precise measurement of the refractive error can be made with trial lenses and a focimeter.

Simultantest (Zeiss (Oberkochen))

The Simultantest is a small trial case accessory that is used subjectively to refine both the sphere and cylindrical components of a refraction. It fits into a trial frame and allows the patient to see the effects of the plus and minus sphere simultaneously, or to see the two flipped positions of the crossed cylinder. A diagram of the optics of the instrument is given in *Figure 9.1*.

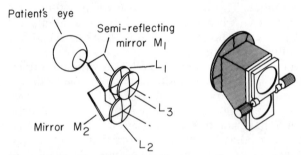

Figure 9.1. The Simultans device. The power of lens L_1 is +0.25; that of L_2 is plano/−0.50 ax 90; that of L_3 is +0.25/−0.50 ax 180

The lens L_3 can be flipped to cover either the top aperture or the bottom one. The mirrors M_1 (semi-reflecting) and M_2 are positioned so as to give two images of the same object to the patient. The first image is seen through L_1, while the second image is seen through L_2 (L_3 can be combined with either of these lenses). When L_3 is combined with L_1, as shown in the diagram, then the first image is seen through a combined power of +0.25/−0.50 ax 90 and the second image through +0.25/−0.50 ax 180. (Axes other than 90 and 180 can be obtained by rotating the instrument.) When L_3 is flipped to cover the lower aperture, the first image is seen through a +0.25 DS and the second image through a combined power of −0.25 DS.

To refine the sphere component of the correction

Lens L_3 is combined with L_2. The patient is asked whether the upper or lower image is clearer. If the upper is clearer, negative power is added and vice versa. Care must be taken to control accommodation as with any other subjective test.

To refine the axis of any cylindrical component

The cylindrical lens is assumed to be already in the trial frame. Lens L_3 is combined with L_1. Set the axis of the Simultantest at 45 degrees to the axis of the cylinder already present. The patient or optometrist then rotates the cylinder and Simultantest until both images appear equally clear.

To refine the power of any cylindrical component

Lens L_3 is combined with L_1. Put the Simultantest along the axis of the cylinder. If the upper image is clearer, then negative cylindrical power is added.

There are two important points to be made about the Simultantest. First, its optical system reduces the contrast of the target, which can make it difficult for a patient to judge which is the clearest image. Second, although the name of the instrument implies that the targets are viewed simultaneously, this is not strictly correct. The two images are separated by approximately 5 degrees and a small eye movement is necessary in order to change fixation from one target image to the other.

Auto Cross (Topcon)

The Auto Cross is fitted by Topcon to their VT-SD refracting unit. It consists of an opaque carrier disc that contains two apertures, each of which contains a 3 D prism (bases towards each other) and a cross cylinder. The cross cylinder in one aperture is at 90 degrees to that in the other. When looking through the device, the patient sees two images of a distant target, one through each of the cross cylinders. The axis and power of any cylindrical component is found in the same way as that described for the Simultantest. The Auto Cross is linked to the refracting unit and rotates with the cylindrical lenses of the unit. To check sphere power, Topcon have produced a second device in which the cross cylinders have been replaced by red and green filters. This attachment operates in the same way as a normal duochrome.

References

BENNETT, A. G. (1966). Trial case lenses ancient and modern. *Ophthalmic Optician*, **6**, 964
BRITISH STANDARD (1959). *Ophthalmic Trial Case Lenses*, BS 3162. British Standards Institution, London
DE ZENG, H. L. (1908). *Lens System for Measuring the Refraction of the Eye*. US patent 886-770
KELLNER, G. A. H. (1918). *Ophthalmic Test Lens Set*. US patent 1 265 671
LANG, M. M. and MARG, E. (1975). Computer-assisted eye examinations IV. 'Additive' lens systems in eye refractors. *American Journal of Optometry and Physiological Optics*, **52**, 533
MARG, E. (1980). *Computer-Assisted Eye Examination*. San Francisco Press, San Francisco
TILLYER, E. D. (1923). *Trial Lens*. US patent 1 455 457

10

Visual acuity instrumentation

Introduction

Certainly the most commonly performed measurement taken in optometric practice is that of the visual acuity. This measurement is normally undertaken with the aid of a test chart. The simplicity of the test chart must not be allowed to cloud one's judgement of its value as a technique for measuring visual acuity. It is the one test of acuity that satisfies practically all the requirements of the optometrist. As a test, it is easily understood by almost the whole population. It is capable of providing an estimate of the acuity within a very short period of time and it is sensitive enough to pick up the amount of blur induced by a 0.25 D lens. While other tests can provide the optometrist with a more accurate measure of the acuity, which may in itself be important in the recognition of certain abnormal conditions, this increased accuracy is redundant as far as routine refraction is concerned.

In this chapter, I describe the major design parameters of modern test charts. Following this I describe chart projectors and projection screens. At the end of the chapter both semi-automated and objective methods of measuring visual acuity are discussed. This latter topic is of special interest to the optometrist because it can provide a means of measuring the acuity in that small percentage of the population that either cannot or chooses not to give reliable results with the test chart.

Test charts

Test charts are designed to give the practitioner a quick estimation of a patient's visual acuity. They are based upon a measurement of the minimum separable, although the majority are in fact measuring the minimum recognizable.

Test chart acuities are usually specified as Snellen fractions in which the denominator equals the distance at which the critical detail of the symbol subtends 1 min of arc and the numerator equals the testing distance. For example, the Snellen fraction 6/9 means that the critical detail of the symbol subtends 1 min of arc at 9 m and that the testing distance was 6 m. In Europe, these two distances are specified in metres and in America they are specified in feet. The Americans have also chosen 20 ft as the standard testing distance, while in Europe it is 6 m. Test chart acuities can be expressed in many other ways – for example, as the decimal equivalent of the Snellen fraction. The Snellen fraction has, however, become the standard clinical technique for specifying the visual acuity. For a review of some of the other techniques, the reader is referred to Borish (1970).

Types of symbol

The majority of currently produced test charts use non-serif letters constructed within a 5 × 4 or a 5 × 5 box. The critical detail of all these letters is taken as the unit size of the construction box square (*see Figure 10.1*). One of the problems of using letters is that they are not all equally

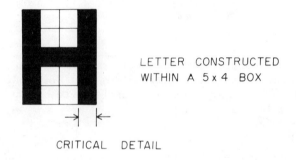

LETTER CONSTRUCTED
WITHIN A 5 x 4 BOX

CRITICAL DETAIL

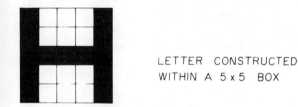

LETTER CONSTRUCTED
WITHIN A 5 x 5 BOX

Figure 10.1. Two styles of symbol often found in modern test charts

legible. Sheard (1921) calculated the relative acuity required for the perception of letters of the same size (*see Table 10.1*). From his findings, he divided the letters into four groups of varying difficulty and suggested that in order to overcome the legibility problem at least one letter from each group should be included on each line. The British Standard (1968) test chart solves the problem of unequal legibility by including only those letters that have approximately equal legibility, i.e. D E F H N P R U V Z*.

* These letters are of equal legibility when they are constructed in the non-serif form within a 5 × 4 box (Woodruff, 1947). Sheard's work was based upon serif letters.

Two other types of test chart commonly found in optometric practice utilize either a series of Es (5 × 5 construction) or a series of Cs (5 × 5 construction), arranged such that the stems of the Es or gaps in the Cs point in different directions. The patient's task is to report the orientation of the letter. These charts are valuable in assessing the acuity of illiterate patients and can successfully be used with the majority of children over the

TABLE 10.1. The relative acuity of different letters (After Sheard, 1921)

Letter	Visual acuity	Letter	Visual acuity	Letter	Visual acuity
L	0.70	Y	0.80	E	0.85
T	0.74	F	0.81	R	0.85
V	0.78	P	0.81	S	0.88
U	0.79	D	0.81	G	0.89
C	0.79	Z	0.84	H	0.92
O	0.80	N	0.84	B	1.00

age of 3½ years. Because of the uniformity of symbol design, these charts give a slightly better estimation of a patient's acuity than the more conventional letter chart. The preference for the letter chart is based upon the speed with which a result can be obtained.

Progression of letter sizes

The progression of letter sizes from one line to the next has been found in the majority of charts to most closely approximate a geometrical progression of letter size, i.e. the letters on each successive line are r times larger than those of the previous line, where r is a constant.

TABLE 10.2. The progression of letter sizes in the British Standard test chart, in a geometrical progression of 1.43, and in the Bailey–Lovie chart

British Standard test chart	Geometrical progression (r = 1.43)	Bailey–Lovie
6/60	6/60	20/200
6/36	6/42	20/160
6/24	6/30	20/125
6/18	6/21	20/100
6/12	6/15	20/80
6/9	6/10	20/63
6/6	6/7	20/50
6/5	6/5	20/40
		20/32
		20/25
		20/20
		20/16
		20/12.5
		20/10

Table 10.2 gives the step sizes of the British Standard test chart and the test chart recommended by Bailey and Lovie (1976). For comparison with the British Standard test chart, a geometrical progression with $r = 1.43$ is also included. The chart recommended by Bailey and Lovie (1976) has been designed to follow a geometrical progression of 1.26 or 0.1 log units. This progression has also been recommended by Green (1867) and Sloan (1959) and has been accepted by the International Council of Ophthalmology Committee on Optotypes (Ogle, 1953). As can be seen from *Table 10.2*, the Bailey–Lovie chart has a much greater number of lines than the British Standard chart. A problem with having such a large number of lines is that the difference in legibility between different letters often results in a patient being able to read certain letters two or more lines below the line in which he starts to make mistakes. The fine gradations of acuity encountered with this type of chart are therefore not really practical for charts that use symbols of differing legibility.

The spacing between symbols

When the symbols on a chart are placed close to one another, a phenomenon known as contour interaction occurs, which reduces the recorded test chart acuity. To overcome this problem, Bailey and Lovie (1976) recommended that the separation of the letters should be equal to the letter width and that each row should be separated by the height of the letters in the smaller row. The British Standard (1968) test chart contains no recommendation about letter spacing other than that they should be evenly spaced and that the rows should be separated by at least 20 mm.

The width of the interaction zone increases with low acuity. For this reason amblyopes often record higher acuities on charts where only a single letter exists on each line.

Test chart luminances

The Committee on Standards of the American Optometric Association recommends that the luminance of the test chart be 10–15 foot lamberts ($34–51 \text{ cd/m}^2$), while the British Standard (1968) gives a recommended minimum for new test charts of 150 cd/m^2. While this difference is large, *Figure 10.2* demonstrates that it has only a small effect upon the measured acuity. This graph of König's data shows that a test chart luminance of 15 cd/m^2 would yield a decimal acuity of approximately 1.55, while a test chart luminance of 150 cd/m^2 would yield a decimal acuity of approximately 1.70. Conversion into Snellen fractions gives values of 20/12.9 and 20/11.8, respectively, i.e. less than one line on the Bailey–Lovie chart.

Contrast of letters

Sloan (1951) has shown that, providing the contrast of the letters is above 84 per cent, variations have a negligible effect upon the acuity. While this

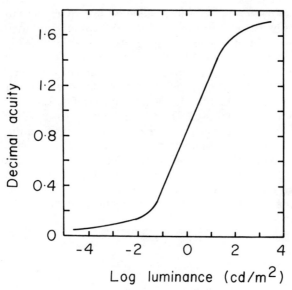

Figure 10.2. Variation of the visual acuity with luminance.
Data of König. After Le Grand (1967)

level of contrast is relatively easy to obtain with internally illuminated test charts, it is much more difficult to obtain with projected charts, where any background illumination on the screen reduces the contrast (*see* Chart projector screens, pp. 197–198).

Chart projectors

Rather than use a printed chart, which is either internally or externally illuminated, many practitioners have opted for a projected chart. The main advantage of a projection system is the large range of charts that can be incorporated into the projector.

Chart projectors are optically identical to slide projectors. The filament of the bulb is imaged at or close to the projection lens system (*see Figure 10.3*). This arrangement maximizes the amount of light which passes through the projection lens and keeps the illumination of the screen even. The projection lens system is usually composed of two lenses, both of which can be independently moved back and forth. This arrangement allows the optometrist to alter the magnification of the chart to the correct value for the projection distance used.

The better, and more expensive, chart projectors contain the slides within a sealed unit in order to keep them clean. They also tend to have a more convenient method of chart control. For a review of the facilities found in several of the currently marketed instruments, the reader is referred to Sasieni (1979).

Augsberger, Sheedy and Schoessler (1979) have compared the intensities of four common chart projectors (the American Optical Project-O-Chart, the Bausch and Lomb Compact, the Biotronics Remote Access and the American Optical Custom Automatic). They found that the luminance of a test plate placed in the beam of each projector varied from approximately 15 cd/m^2 for the American Optical Project-O-Chart to over 60 cd/m^2 for the American Optical Custom Automatic, with the Bausch and Lomb and the Biotronics instruments giving just over 20 and just under 30 cd/m^2. This large range of intensities reflects the lack of any standardization of chart projectors. Its importance as far as the recording of visual acuity is concerned is, however, only slight. It can be seen from *Figure 10.2* that by increasing the intensity of the chart from 10 to 100 cd/m^2 the

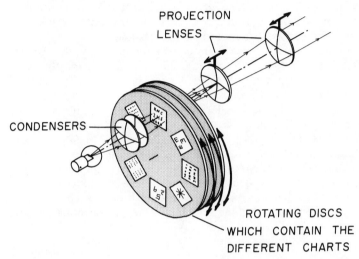

Figure Figure 10.3. An isometric diagram showing the optics of a chart projector

decimal acuity improves from just under 1.4 to 1.6, which in Snellen notation would be 20/14.3 to 20/12.5 – i.e. approximately one line on the Bailey–Lovie recommended chart (*see Table 10.2*). The four-fold difference in intensities between the two American Optical projectors would therefore produce less than one line difference between the recorded acuities.

It should be remembered while discussing chart projectors that the actual intensity of the chart is dependent upon both the intensity of the projector and the reflective properties of the screen.

Chart projector screens

The majority of screens used with chart projectors specularly reflect the incident illumination in order to retain any polarization. An unwanted side effect of this is that the intensity of a projected image varies with viewing angle, being at a maximum when the screen is viewed along the primary angle of reflectance. Augsberger, Sheedy and Schoessler (1979) measured how the luminance of five different screens varied with the viewing angle. The American Optical screen was found to be the most sensitive to changes in viewing angle; its luminance fell by approximately 75 per cent when the viewing angle was 20 degrees off the primary reflectance angle. This high sensitivity to viewing angle can be considered in two ways: as undesirable, because it means that the positioning of the screen, projector and patient is fairly critical, and as advantageous, because it means that the reflectance from the screen is more specular. The more highly specular the reflectance is, the greater will be both the intensity of the image and the percentage of polarization retained after reflection. The results of other measurements taken by Augsberger, Sheedy and Schoessler (1979) verify this. The American Optical screen was found to have the highest luminance of all the screens tested and to retain the greatest percentage of polarization.

All projection systems need to overcome the problem of maintaining high contrast values in rooms which contain some ambient illumination. While examinations can be conducted in a darkened room, this is not comfortable for the patient and is not recommended by the British Standard (1968), which suggests that the minimum background illumination be equal to 10 per cent of that of the chart. Any background illumination that falls on the screen will reduce the contrast of the symbols. In an unpublished study by Schoessler and Uniacke (1979), it was found that while the contrast levels in 20 different consulting rooms were, on average, 99 per cent with the room light off, this level fell to 84.6 per cent with two ceiling lights on. The effect of room lighting upon the contrast of the projected image is dependent upon the specular reflecting properties of the screen. The more highly specular screens will be affected less by room illumination, provided that the room lights are positioned such that their primary angle of reflectance from the screen is as far away as possible from the patient's viewing angle.

Baylor Video Acuity Tester

A novel type of test chart that has only recently been developed is the Baylor Video Acuity Tester. As the name implies, this test chart is based upon a television monitor. The display on the monitor is controlled by a keyboard which allows the optometrist to:

1. Select letters at any one of 14 different sizes;
2. Step up or down to the next size of letter;
3. Select Snellen or illiterate E targets;
4. Change the letters or orientation of the E without changing the size;
5. Use single or multiple displays of up to five letters;
6. Present the letters as either black on white or white on black;
7. Insert filters for duochrome testing;
8. Zoom the letter sizes either up or down;
9. Store, in a small memory, the visual acuity of the patient.

On the negative side:

1. The instrument is currently restricted in the types of character that it can display to those that do not have diagonal elements;

2. The instrument cannot be used as a replacement for conventional test charts because it does not contain features such as fan charts, cross cylinders targets and Mallett units;
3. It is only capable of displaying one line of letters at a time. This means that the process of establishing the initial visual acuity of a patient is more tedious for the optometrist who continually has to change the display.

Automatic acuity measurement

In 1970, Crossman, Goodeve and Marg devised an automatic technique for recording a patient's visual acuity which utilized a small computer, a random access slide projector and a joystick lever. The computer would present to the patient a slide which contained a single Landolt C and then wait for the patient to respond by pushing the lever in the direction of the gap in the C. Depending upon the patient's response, the computer would then present either a smaller or larger symbol. At the end of a series of measurements, the computer would then calculate the patient's acuity and print out the result. This technique of establishing the acuity has been adopted in the Baylor Acuity Meter. The Baylor instrument consists of a small display unit into which the patient looks and a control box which contains all the electronic logic.

Decker *et al.* (1975) have both described and evaluated the Baylor instrument and state that the results correlate well with those obtained with a standard Snellen chart and that it can be used successfully on children as young as 4 years of age. The disadvantages of this instrument are that it is relatively expensive and that it takes longer than an equivalent letter chart measurement.

Objective determination of visual acuity

To be able to objectively record the visual acuity of a patient has been the goal of many clinicians for some considerable time. The rewards for success in this field include the ability to measure visual acuity in young children, in illiterates and in the mentally handicapped. There have, over the years, been a considerable number of attempts to develop a reliable objective test. Voipio (1961) has classified these into four groups:

1. Methods based upon evoking an oscillatory eye movement;
2. Methods based upon evoking optokinetic nystagmus;
3. Methods based upon arresting optokinetic nystagmus;
4. Methods based upon the galvanic skin response.

Methods based upon evoking an oscillatory eye movement

The originator of this technique was Goldmann (1943) and it can best be understood by referring to *Figure 10.4*, which is a diagram of Goldmann's apparatus. The central, coarse-chequered pattern is made to oscillate from side to side in front of a much finer chequered pattern, the elements of which are beyond the resolving power of the eye. If the patient is able to resolve the oscillating chequered pattern then the eyes will follow it and produce an oscillating eye movement of the same frequency as that of the pattern. If the central pattern is beyond the resolving power of the eye, then the patient will seen an even, grey area, the central pattern blending into the finer background. Under these circumstances the patient's eye will fail to produce the oscillatory eye movement.

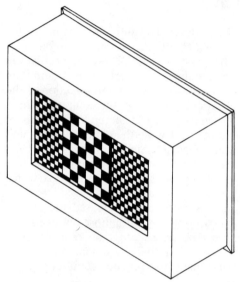

Figure 10.4. Goldmann's apparatus for the objective measurement of visual acuity

The patient is told to look at the central part of the chequered pattern and the examiner views the eye through a magnifier in order to establish whether or not it is moving at the correct frequency. The patient is moved either closer to or further from the instrument in order to alter the angular subtence of the central pattern and obtain a quantitative measure of the visual acuity.

There are two commercially available pieces of equipment based upon the Goldmann technique. The first of these was developed by Millodot, Miller and Jernigan (1973) who attached the oscillating target to a Biometrics eye movement recorder and replaced the chequered pattern with a series of square wave gratings of different spatial frequencies (*see Figure 10.5*). The practitioner instructs the patient to view the oscillating grating and monitors the eye movements with the recorder. The finest grating with which oscillatory eye movements of the correct temporal frequency can be seen is taken as a measure of the patient's acuity.

The second commercially available piece of equipment that falls into this category is the Catford visual acuity device (*see Figure 10.6*). This instrument utilizes a single oscillating black dot as a target, the diameter of

OSCILLATING   GRATING

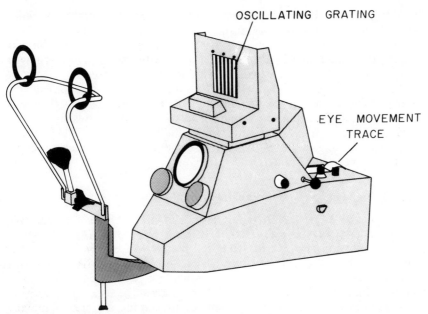

EYE   MOVEMENT
TRACE

Figure 10.5. Millodot's objective acuity apparatus attached to the Biometrics eye movement recorder (Millodot, Miller and Jernigan, 1973)

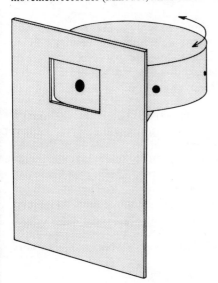

Figure 10.6. The Catford visual acuity device (Catford and Oliver, 1973)

which is reduced, in discrete steps, until the examiner can no longer detect any oscillatory eye movements. The smallest dot size with which oscillatory movements can be detected is taken as the measure of the acuity. Each dot is marked with the equivalent 6 m Snellen acuity.

Atkinson *et al.* (1981) have, in an evaluation of this instrument, pointed out that the detection of a small spot is primarily a test of contrast detection rather than visual resolution. When they compared Landolt C acuities with those from the Catford device in a group of normal subjects with either induced or naturally occurring refractive errors, they found that the Catford instrument grossly overestimated the Landolt C acuity. Subjects with the equivalent of 6/24 acuity as measured with the Landolt Cs showed the equivalent of 6/6 acuity with the Catford acuity device.

Khan, Chen and Frenkel (1976) also reported that the objectively recorded acuity with the Catford instrument was considerably higher than the conventionally recorded Snellen acuity. They did, however, find a fairly good correlation between its results and those of a standard Snellen chart. This finding indicates that the instrument could give fairly reliable results if it were recalibrated.

Methods based upon evoking optokinetic nystagmus

Optokinetic nystagmus (OKN) is a particular pattern of eye movements seen when a person views a resolvable moving target. It consists of a series of slow, following movements separated by fast, refixatory saccades that move the eye in the opposite direction to the pursuit movements. This pattern of eye movements is often seen when a person looks out of the window of a moving train. The OKN response can be used to objectively measure the visual acuity of a patient by presenting a series of moving targets of gradually increasing spatial frequency. When the spatial frequency of the target exceeds the resolving power of the eye, then the OKN response will stop.

A large number of researchers have reported techniques that utilize the OKN response to objectively measure the visual acuity (*see* Pearson, 1966, for a review). The majority of them used black and white chequered or striped patterns which were gradually moved across the visual field of the patient while the clinician examined the eyes for OKN.

The only commercially available piece of equipment that utilizes this technique is the OKN drum. This instrument consists of a rotating drum on the outside of which is painted a black and white grating. The drum is rotated in front of the patient's eyes while the practitioner looks at the eyes for an OKN response. As a measure of visual acuity, this test is extremely crude as the size and spatial frequency of the grating is such that OKN can be elicited in patients with very low acuities. The high correlations between Snellen acuity and the OKN technique that have been reported by several researchers have been obtained with instruments that can produce high spatial frequency gratings which cannot be resolved by patients with low acuity. The value of the OKN drum is in establishing whether or not very young children can see.

Methods based upon arresting optokinetic nystagmus

This group again uses OKN, only in a slightly different manner. If a patient is able to view a stationary object within a moving (OKN stimulating) field, then his OKN will be suppressed. Voipio (1961) and Voipio and Hyvarinen (1966) have used this phenomenon to develop an objective technique for recording the visual acuity. Their apparatus generates a pattern that is composed of two elements which, when combined, appear as in *Figure*

10.7. The first element is a moving saw-tooth pattern which is capable of eliciting an OKN response in patients with very low acuities. The second element is a diffuse grey pattern in the centre of which is a black and white horizontal grating. When the grating is out of focus it blends into the grey background and cannot be resolved.

When measuring the acuity of a patient with this apparatus, the central grating is initially set out of focus with the result that the patient exhibits an OKN response to the moving saw-tooth pattern. It is then gradually brought into focus while the practitioner views the patient's eye or a trace of the eye movements (Voipio and Hyvarinen, 1966). If the OKN is seen to

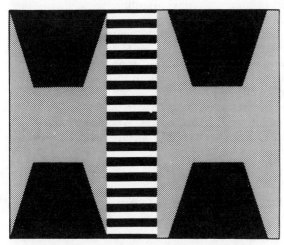

Figure 10.7. The target pattern used by Voipio for the objective measurement of visual acuity

stop then it is taken that the patient can resolve the grating. By using gratings of different spatial frequencies, the visual acuity of the patient is measured.

Currently, there are no commercially available pieces of equipment based upon this technique, even though it has been shown by Voipio (Voipio, 1961; Voipio and Hyvarinen, 1966) to correlate very well with Snellen acuity.

Methods based upon the galvanic skin response

This technique, which has only been described by one researcher (Wagner, 1950), requires a patient to be conditioned to a particular target (e.g. a Snellen letter) by giving him a small electric shock every time the target is shown. Eventually, a measured anticipatory potential can be recorded from the skin every time the letter is shown. By altering the size of letters, after conditioning, the resolving power of the eye can be established.

Summary

The most common technique for assessing the validity of an objective acuity device is to correlate its measurement of acuity with those from a standard Snellen test in a group of normal patients. A problem with using the correlation coefficient in this way is that the value of the coefficient is dependent upon the sample size and range of acuities within the sample. Strictly, techniques can only be compared with this statistic when they have been used on equivalent populations. As this is certainly not the case for the majority of reported values, the reader should be careful in making any judgements about the efficacy of a particular test or group of tests solely on its correlation coefficient.

Although these tests are all objective, this does not mean that they can be reliably used on all segments of the population. The problems of getting very young children, for instance, to pay attention to a small, high frequency grating are such that a negative result with the first three tests described above does not necessarily mean that the acuity is low. Problems can also arise if patients intentionally try to foil the tests by either viewing to one side of the stimulating field in tests that rely upon the eliciting of eye movements or by ignoring the stationary grating in tests which rely upon the arresting of OKN.

In summary, when a positive result is obtained with these tests it tells the practitioner that the patient can resolve the grating. When a negative result is obtained it means that either the test was unsuccessful or that the patient's acuity is low.

References

ATKINSON, J., BRADDICK, O., PIMM-SMITH, E., AYLING, L. and SAWYER, R. (1981). Does the Catford drum give an accurate assessment of acuity? *British Journal of Ophthalmology*, **65**, 652

AUGSBERGER, A., SHEEDY, J. E. and SCHOESSLER, J. P. (1979). Reflectance of visual acuity screens. *American Journal of Optometry and Physiological Optics*, **56**, 531

BAILEY, I. L. and LOVIE, J. E. (1976). New design principles for visual acuity letter charts. *American Journal of Optometry and Physiological Optics*, **53**, 740

BORISH, I. (1970). *Clinical Refraction*. The Professional Press, Chicago

BRITISH STANDARD (1968). *Test Charts for Determining Distance Visual Acuity*, BS 4274. British Standards Institution, London

CATFORD, G. V. and OLIVER, A. (1973). Development of visual acuity. *Archives of Diseases in Childhood*, **48**, 47

CROSSMAN, E. R. F. W., GOODEVE, P. J. and MARG, E. (1970). A computer based automatic method for determining visual acuity. *American Journal of Optometry and Archives of the American Academy of Optometry*, **47**, 344

DECKER, T. A., KUETHER, C. L., WILLIAMS, R. E. and LOGAR, N. D. (1975). A semi-automated instrument for determination of acuity threshold. *Archives of Ophthalmology*, **93**, 841

GOLDMANN, H. (1943). Objective Sehacharfenbestimmung. *Ophthalmologica*, **105**, 204

GREEN, J. (1867). Cited in Bailey and Lovie (1976)

KHAN, S. G., CHEN, K. F. and FRENKEL, M. (1976). Subjective and objective visual acuity testing techniques. *Archives of Ophthalmology*, **94**, 2086

KÖNIG (1897). Cited in Le Grand (1967)

LE GRAND, Y. (1967). *Form and Space Vision*. Translated by M. Millodot and G. Heath. Indiana University Press, Bloomington

OGLE, K. N. (1953). On the problem of an international nomenclature for designating visual acuity. *American Journal of Ophthalmology*, **36**, 909

MILLODOT, M., MILLER, D. and JERNIGAN, M. E. (1973). Evaluation of an objective acuity device. *Archives of Ophthalmology*, **90**, 449

PEARSON, R. M. (1966). The objective determination of vision and visual acuity. *British Journal of Physiological Optics*, **23**, 107

SASIENI, L. (1979). A guide to chart projectors. *Optician*, **177**, Jan 12th, 9

SCHOESSLER, J. P. and UNIACKE, C. A. (1979). Cited in Augsberger, Sheedy and Schoessler (1979)

SHEARD, C. (1921). Some factors affecting visual acuity. *American Journal of Physiological Optics,* **2,** 168

SLOAN, L. L. (1951). Measurement of visual acuity. A critical review. *Archives of Ophthalmology,* **45,** 704

SLOAN, L. L. (1959). New charts for the measurment of visual acuity at far and near distances. *American Journal of Ophthalmology,* **48,** 807

VOIPIO, H. (1961). The objective measurement of visual acuity by arresting optokinetic nystagmus without change in illumination. *Acta Ophthalmologica,* **66,** (Suppl), 1

VOIPIO, H. and HYVARINEN, L. (1966). Objective measurement of visual acuity by arresovisography. *Archives of Ophthalmology,* **75,** 799

WAGNER, H. N. (1950). Cited by Pearson (1966)

WOODRUFF, E. W. (1947). Cited by Borish (1970)

11

Lens checking equipment

Introduction

The practitioner requires lens checking equipment in order to both verify his own prescriptions when returned from the laboratory and to measure the prescriptions supplied by other practitioners. Ideally, the optometrist should be able to verify or measure all the parameters specified in a lens order. While it is possible to do this with current lens checking equipment for spectacle lenses, it is not possible to do this for contact lenses. Currently, there exists no satisfactory way of measuring the peripheral curves of hard contact lenses and no reliable, non destructive way of measuring hard or soft lens materials.

The lens checking equipment that does exist can be divided into three basic categories according to the parameter that it was originally designed to measure. These parameters are:

1. The measurement of vertex power. This measurement is normally made with a focimeter (lensmeter) although it can also be made with a set of trial lenses, utilizing the technique of neutralization. The latter technique is more time consuming and less precise than the former;
2. The measurement of radii of curvature. This type of measurement is especially important in contact lens work where incorrect radii can lead to unsuccessful fits;
3. The measurement of thickness. Again, this parameter is of special importance to the contact lens practitioner. In soft contact lens fitting, the thickness of the lens is an important parameter in controlling the amount of oxygen that reaches the cornea.

In this chapter, lens checking equipment is grouped according to the parameters outlined above. The chapter begins with a description of the focimeter (lensmeter). I then go on to describe radius measuring devices and conclude with thickness measuring devices. In each group, the measurement of spectacle lenses, hard contact lenses and soft contact lenses is considered.

The focimeter

The focimeter, or lensmeter, was originally designed to measure the vertex power and optical centration of spectacle lenses. It can, however, and with only slight modification, also be used to measure the vertex power of hard and soft contact lenses and the back central optic radius of hard contact lenses.

Optical principles and basic construction

Nearly all the commercially available instruments are based upon the same optical construction (*see Figure 11.1*). The lens being measured is placed against a stop between a standard lens and an afocal telescope. A target on the other side of the standard lens is then moved back and forth until a

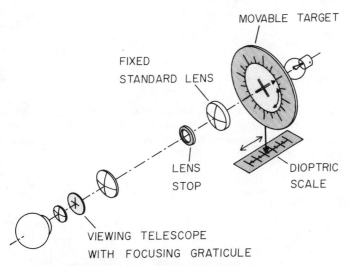

Figure 11.1. An isometric diagram of the optics of the focimeter

clear image of the target is seen by the observer through the telescope. The lens stop is positioned such that its centre falls at the anterior focal point of the standard lens. This arrangement ensures that the dioptric scale is linear and that the image size of the target is not affected by the power of the lens being measured. The same principle is utilized in the Badal optometer (*see* Chapter 8).

The optical theory upon which the focimeter is based is shown in *Figure 11.2*. Using Newton's relationship, i.e. $xx' = -f'^2$, we can see that:

$$xx' = -xf'v = -f'_0{}^2$$
$$f'v = f'_0{}^2/x$$
$$F'v = F_0{}^2x$$

Since the power of the standard lens, F_0, is a constant for any given focimeter, the back-vertex power of the lens being measured is proportional to the distance x.

The range of powers that can be measured with a focimeter is determined by the power of the standard lens, the maximum measurable positive power being slightly less than the standard lens power, which in most focimeters is between +22 D and +27 D. As the power of the standard lens is increased, the amount of target movement per dioptre of vergence decreases. In an instrument with a 27.00 D lens, the target would move 1.37 mm for every dioptre of vergence, while the target of an

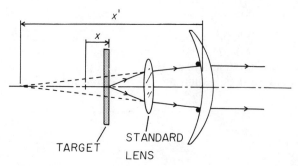

Figure 11.2. The arrangement of the focimeters optical elements

instrument with a 22 D standard lens would move 2.06 mm for every dioptre of vergence. Because of this relationship, the manufacturers of focimeters often have to compromise between accuracy and range when designing a particular instrument.

Sources of error

Eyepiece focusing

Prior to using a focimeter, it is important to focus the eyepiece of the telescope such that a clear, sharp image of the target is seen when the vergence of light incident upon the objective of the telescope is zero. The eyepiece is focused by setting the focimeter reading to zero and then screwing the eyepiece in, from its outmost position, until the target is sharply focused. Failure to focus the eyepiece can cause errors in excess of 1 D.

Position of the lens vertex

The calibration of focimeters is based upon the assumption that the back surface of the lens is coincident with the lens stop. With highly convex or concave lenses, the position of the lens will be slightly behind or in front of this stop (*see Figure 11.3*). Bennett (1968) calculates that the error due to the shift in vertex position may reach 0.12 D for a 20 D spectacle lens. To overcome this problem, Essilor have incorporated a non-linear scale within their Frontofocimeter that compensates for the changing position of the lens vertex with changes in lens power. While this improves the accuracy of this instrument in the measurement of the back-vertex power of spectacle

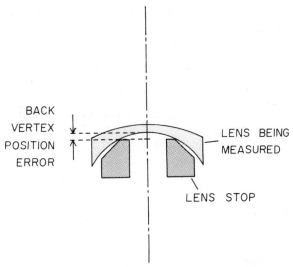

Figure 11.3. The back-vertex position error that occurs with high-power lenses

lenses, it can lead to problems when the instrument is used to measure front-vertex powers.

The back-vertex position error increases when the focimeter is used to measure the power of contact lenses. Because of the steep back radii of these lenses, this error may exceed 0.25 D. The size of this error can be reduced by decreasing the lens stop diameter from its normal value of approximately 6 mm.

Spherical aberration in contact lenses

The high curvature of contact lenses means that the spherical aberration at a point 3 mm from the optical centre can exceed 2 D on a −10 D lens. If the back-vertex power of a contact lens were measured with the normal 6 mm diameter stop, then the image quality would be poor and the final result, assuming the operator adjusted for the best focus, would be different from the axial back-vertex power. Reducing the stop diameter to 3 mm means that the focimeter will be measuring within 1.5 mm of the lens' optical centre, where the spherical aberration on the same −10 D lens will not exceed 0.5 D.

Filter

Many focimeters have a green filter over the target pattern. Because the power of a lens is defined by reference to light of wavelength 587.6 nm, a small error (not exceeding 0.1 D) can occur on high-power spectacle lenses.

Drum backlash

Some focimeters have the dioptric scale attached to a drum wheel which alters the position of the target through a rack and pinion arrangement.

Any backlash in the gearing can result in errors between the true dioptric position of the target and the drum scale. This problem can be overcome by attaching the scale to the target and then arranging for the scale to be viewed through an eyepiece.

Quality of the standard lens

One of the parameters that affects the accuracy of a focimeter is the quality of its standard lens. Any aberrations in this lens will affect the image quality and thus the accuracy of setting. It can be seen from *Figure 11.4*

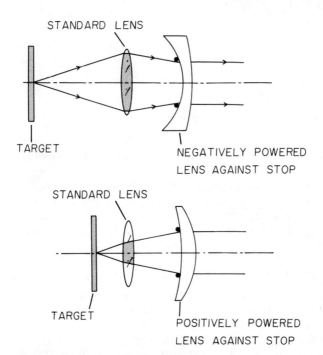

Figure 11.4. The area of the standard lens used varies with the power of the lens being measured

that the area of the standard lens used varies with the power of the lens being measured. The more negative the lens, the greater the area. This means that any aberrations of the standard lens will be more noticeable when the focimeter is used to check lenses of high negative power. This finding leads to a simple means of comparing the quality of standard lenses in different focimeters. The optometrist should compare the quality of the targets image when measuring the same high-power negative lens.

Projection focimeters

Some focimeters have replaced the telescope arrangement with a projection device (*see Figures 11.5 and 11.6*). The main advantage of this arrangement is that it overcomes any errors due to the operator failing to focus the eyepiece correctly and/or due to accommodation during the measurement. Projection focimeters are particularly valuable in clinics where a large number of people will be using the same instrument as it saves each operator from having to focus the eyepiece every time the instrument is used. Projection focimeters are also useful for teaching purposes as they allow more than one operator to view the target at the

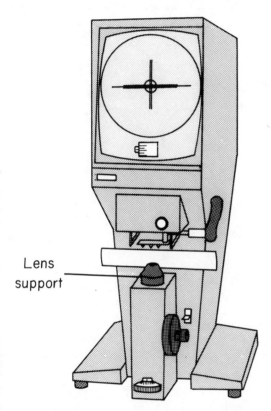

Lens
support

Figure 11.5. Projection focimeter (Nikon)

same time. Finally, it is claimed that they are less fatiguing. A survey of many of the currently produced projection focimeters has been written by Woodcock (1980).

Use of the focimeter to measure soft lens power

Sarver *et al.* (1973) describe a technique whereby the back-vertex power of a soft contact lens can be measured with a focimeter. The lens is surface dried, by blotting with a lint-free tissue, before being placed on the focimeter lens rest. Measurements have to be made fairly rapidly or else the lens starts to dry out, which results in a distortion of the focimeter image.

To overcome the problem of drying out, Poster (1971) recommended that the power of a soft lens be measured while it is immersed in a saline filled cell. This technique requires a focimeter of high accuracy (about four times as accurate as that required for spectacle lenses) because the power of a soft lens immersed in saline is considerably less than it would be if measured in air. The focimeter reading taken with the wet cell has to be multiplied by a conversion factor, the value of which is dependent upon the

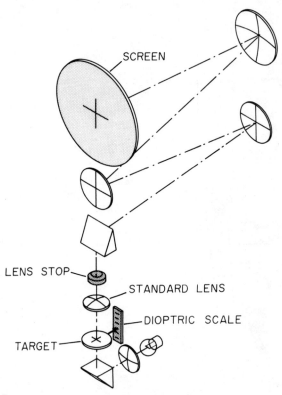

Figure 11.6. The optics of a projection focimeter

refractive index of the lens, its radii of curvature and its thickness (Wichterle, 1965). If we assume that the lens is thin, then the conversion factor can be calulated from equation (11.1) (Harris, Hall and Oye, 1973) which only requires a knowledge of the refractive index of the lens and saline.

$$\text{Conversion factor} = \frac{n_{\text{lens}} - n_{\text{air}}}{n_{\text{lens}} - n_{\text{saline}}} \qquad (11.1)$$

For a soft lens of refractive index 1.43, the conversion factor is calculated to be 4.57.

Both these techniques of measuring soft lens power have been evaluated by Pearson (1980a) who found that the mean of the standard errors of variously powered soft lenses was 0.09 D when measured in air and 0.05 D when measured in saline. When the saline results are multiplied by the conversion factor, using Harris' equation, the mean of the standard errors increases to 0.228 D, a value considerably above that for the measurement in air. The results of Pearson (1980a) indicate, therefore, that a more accurate measurement of soft lens power can be obtained when the lens is measured in air. To obtain accurate results in air, Pearson (1980a) constructed a special lens stop that was capable of supporting the soft lens. Without this special stop, the soft lens invariably flexes under its own weight, making an accurate reading impossible.

Measurement of hard contact lens radii with the focimeter

Sarver and Kerr (1964) have developed an attachment for the focimeter that allows the practitioner to measure the back central optic radius (BCOR) of hard contact lenses. This attachment (*see Figure 11.7*), which is made of the same material as the contact lens (refractive index 1.49), fits over the lens stop of the focimeter and is made so that its convex surface

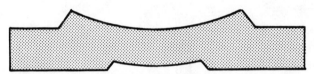

Figure 11.7. Attachment for the measurement of the optic radius of hard contact lenses with a focimeter

lies in the plane of the lens stop. Its concave surface, which supports the lens being measured, is made flatter than the front surface radius of any contact lens that the practitioner is likely to wish to measure. The contact lens is placed, convex surface down, on the concave surface of the attachment or holder and a small amount of fluid (refractive index 1.49) placed between them.

The holder, fluid and contact lens can now be considered as a single thick lens of refractive index 1.49 and centre thickness equal to the thickness of the contact lens plus the thickness of the holder. The radius of curvature of the contact lens can therefore be calculated from equation (11.2)

$$\text{BCOR} = \frac{(1 - n)\,1 + \dfrac{t_1 + t_2}{n}\,(F_v - F_1)}{(F_v - F_1)} \tag{11.2}$$

where:

F_v is the focimeter reading;
F_1 is the power of the holder's front surface;
t_1 is the thickness of the holder;
t_2 is the thickness of the contact lens;
n is the refractive index (1.49)

Sarver and Kerr (1964) state that, with the values chosen by them, each 0.25 D of power is approximately equal to 0.04 mm of radius. In a trial that compared their technique with that of a radiuscope based on Drysdale's principle, the Drysdale radiuscope gave slightly more accurate results.

Automatic focimeters (lensmeters)

Automatic focimeters (lensmeters) do not require any subjective judgement by the operator, whose task is reduced to simply placing the lens on the measuring head and then pressing a button. The power of the lens being measured is then quickly displayed on either a calculator-type display or a small television-type screen. Such instruments can perform measurements very rapidly and can be operated by relatively unskilled staff.

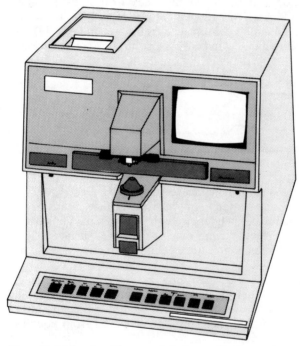

Figure 11.8. Metrolens II automatic focimeter (Rodenstock)

There follows a description of the optics of one of the currently manufactured automatic focimeters, namely the Humphrey Lens Analyzer. Similar instruments are also made by Acuity Systems (The Auto-Lensmeter) and by Rodenstock (Metrolens II) (*Figure 11.8*).

Humphrey Lens Analyzer

To understand how the Humphrey Lens Analyzer operates, we must first consider what happens to an off-axis beam of light when it passes through a spherical spectacle lens. As can be seen from *Figure 11.9*(a) and (b), the beam will be deviated by an extent dependent upon the power of the lens. If we were to place a scale at X, the amount of deviation could be converted into a measure of the lens power. A problem arises with this technique if the lens is not centred correctly as the amount of deviation will vary with the degree of decentration. This problem can be overcome by the use of two beams, as shown in *Figure 11.9*(c) and (d). The difference in the deviation of the two beams gives a measure of the lens power, independently of any decentration. As a bonus, the midpoint of the two beams will give a measure of any prismatic component of the lens at the point being tested.

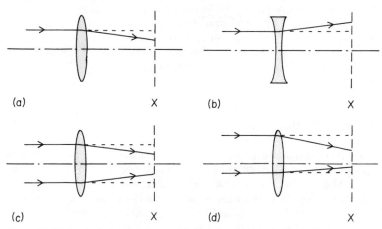

Figure 11.9. The deviation of a beam of light as it passes through a lens

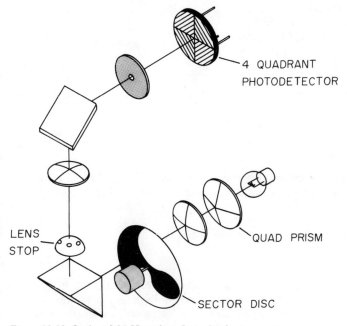

Figure 11.10. Optics of the Humphrey Lens Analyzer

In order to be able to measure cylindrical powers, it is necessary to use at least four beams of light. The resultant pattern will be elliptical, the major and minor axes of which will coincide with the axes of the cylinder under test. The Humphrey Lens Analyzer utilizes four beams of light which are alternately flashed on by the rotation of a sector disc in front of a quad prism (see Figure 11.10). The deviation of each beam is measured by a four quadrant photodetector. This detector will respond to an incident spot of light by giving an electrical signal the magnitude of which is dependent upon the position of the spot. These detectors can typically resolve the position of the spot to within 1/1000 of an inch. The output of the detector is fed into a small computer which processes the information and then displays the spherical, cylindrical and prismatic powers of the lens on a calculator-type display. The computer can also store the information about a particular lens. This is used when checking glazed spectacles to give a measure of both the horizontal and vertical prism at the specified centration distance.

Radius measuring devices

Optometrists routinely need to measure the radius of curvature of a lens surface. A radius of curvature measurement is needed by contact-lens practitioners when they check newly manufactured lenses and by non contact-lens practitioners when they wish to establish the base curve of a spectacle lens. Currently, there are five commonly used techniques for measuring the radius of curvature:

1. By a measurement of the sag;
2. Using Drysdale's principle;
3. By comparison with templates;
4. With the aid of a keratometer;
5. With the aid of a focimeter.

For a description of techniques 4 and 5, the reader is referred to pp. 104–106 and pp. 213–214.

Measurement of the sag

The radius of curvature and power of a surface (if the refractive index is known) can be calculated from a measurement of the sag using equation (11.3).

$$r = \frac{y^2 + s^2}{2s} \tag{11.3}$$

where s is the sag of the lens over a chord diameter $2y$. Equation (11.3) is derived by the application of the theorem of Pythagoras to the triangle ABC of Figure 11.11. The sag principle has been utilized in the spectacle lens spherometer (or lens measure) for many years. It has also been used

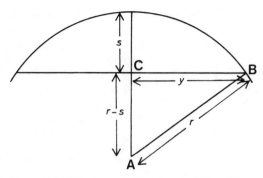

Figure 11.11. The theory behind the calculation of the radius of curvature from a sag measurement

recently in instruments designed to measure the radii of curvature of soft contact lenses.

In the following discussion of instruments that utilize the sag principle, the spectacle lens spherometer is first described, followed by a description of three techniques of measuring the sag of soft contact lenses:

1. By using a central probe;
2. With ultrasound;
3. By measurement from a projected profile.

Spherometer or lens measure

The spherometer (*see Figure 11.12*) is a simple mechanical instrument used to give the power of a spectacle lens surface. Its main use for the

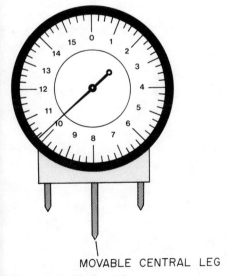

MOVABLE CENTRAL LEG

Figure 11.12. The lens spherometer

optometrist is to check the base curves of spectacle lenses, a measurement that cannot be obtained with the focimeter. The instrument has three pointed legs, the outer two being fixed, while the inner one can slide in and out to make the sag measurement. The inner leg is usually attached to a spring which exerts a small downward pressure on the surface being measured. A rack and pinion mechanism converts the linear position of the central leg into a dial gauge reading.

To convert a sag reading into a dioptric measurement of surface power, it is necessary to know the refractive index of the lens, which is usually 1.530 or 1.523. If the spherometer is used to measure lenses of different refractive index, then the reading should be converted using equation (11.4).

$$\text{Surface power} = \frac{(n-1)}{(n_0-1)} \times \text{spherometer power reading} \qquad (11.4)$$

where n equals the refractive index of the lens being measured and n_0 equals the refractive index used to calibrate the spherometer. Inaccuracies in the spherometer reading occur when the instrument is not held normal to the lens surface and when the legs become worn. Errors due to wear of the legs can be checked by verifying that the dial reads zero when the legs are placed on a flat surface.

One of the disadvantages of the spherometer and all sag measuring devices is that, as yet, no convenient method exists to measure the radii (or power) of toric surfaces.

Soft lens measuring devices that utilize the sag principle and use a central probe

Central probe instruments operate in a similar way to the spectacle lens spherometer. The contact lens is usually supported on the end of a cylinder of known diameter and a central probe is brought up through the cylinder until it contacts the lens. The movement of the probe gives a direct measurement of the sag, which is then converted into a radius measurement.

One of the most basic instruments designed along these lines is the Wöhlk microspherometer (*see Figure 11.13*). The central pin is moved by a calibrated screw mechanism until it first contacts the lens. Recognition of the point of contact is aided by the provision of a small magnifier through which the practitioner can view the lens.

A later instrument, the BC Tronic F (Amisag), replaced the microscope with a simple electronic circuit that turns a light on when the probe first contacts the lens. The electronic circuit operates by measuring the resistance between the central probe and the annulus, which drops rapidly when contact is made because of the electrical conductivity of hydrated soft contact lenses. Similar instruments to the BC Tronic F are made by Neitz (SM 100 Softometer), Kelvin (BCOR Electrogauge) (*see Figure 11.14*) and Rehder (ST-2 sagittal height and thickness gauge). Port (1980) evaluated the accuracy of the Neitz instrument on hard lens materials. He concluded that it was accurate to within ±0.05 mm of radius.

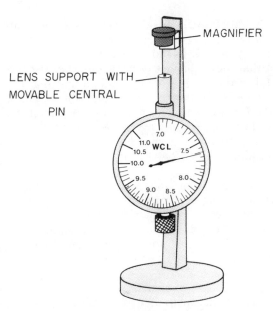

Figure 11.13. The Wöhlk microspherometer

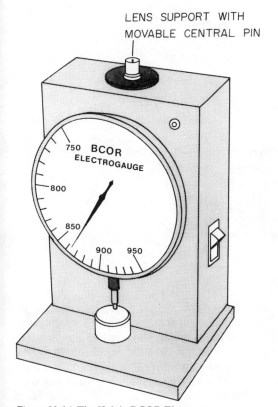

Figure 11.14. The Kelvin BCOR Electrogauge

There are two problems that arise when these instruments are used to measure the radii of soft lenses. First, the lens dries out during the measurement process with the result that its radius changes. Hamano and Kawabe (1978) have shown that these changes occur within the first few minutes of the lens being taken out of its storage medium and that the changes are greater and occur earlier for thin lenses. Second, the weight of the unsupported centre of the lens tends to flatten its radius of curvature. Both of these problems have been successfully overcome in the following three instruments, which are all capable of measuring the sag of a contact lens while it is immersed in saline.

1. Contact Lens Manufacturing Wet Cell Gauge. Operates in a similar way to the Wöhlk microspherometer except that the contact lens is viewed through a compound microscope rather than through a simple magnifier. The standard deviation of a series of 25 measurements of the same soft lens has been given as 0.096 mm, which is better than the Wöhlk microspherometer, but not quite as good as some of the other radius measuring devices (see Table 11.1, p. 226);
2. Kelvin Soft Lens Measuring Gauge. Similar in operation to the BC Tronic F instrument, only in this instrument the central probe is advanced automatically and the result is digitally displayed;

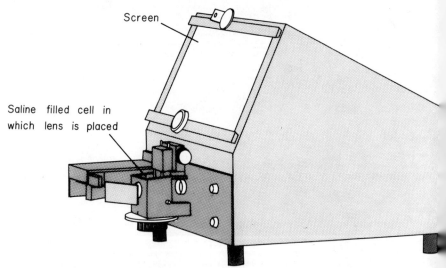

Figure 11.15. The Optimec Contact Lens Analyzer

3. Optimec Contact Lens Analyzer (see Figure 11.15). Operates in the same way as the Wöhlk microspherometer and the Contact Lens Manufacturing Wet Cell Gauge. Rather than viewing the lens through a magnifier or a microscope, however, the practitioner is able to view a projected profile of the lens and central probe. The practitioner advances the probe, via a calibrated screw mechanism, until it is seen to touch the back surface of the lens and then reads off the radius from a scale attached to the knob.

The Optimec Contact Lens Analyzer has been evaluated by Port (1981) who found the standard deviation of a series of measurements to be 0.03 mm for both hard and soft lenses of 40 per cent water content. Port found that the standard deviation of the measurements increased as the water content of the lens increased above 40 per cent. He points out that one of the advantages of this piece of equipment is that it can be used to measure the thickness and diameter of the lens at the same time. Its scale for the measurement of thickness is graduated in 0.02 mm steps, which means that it is not of much value in measuring ultra thin lenses.

In addition to solving the two problems mentioned earlier, the use of a saline bath makes it possible for the practitioner to control the temperature and tonicity of the lens during the measurement process. As both of these parameters affect the lens radius (Loran, 1974; Poster and Skolnik, 1974), more accurate results should be obtained when the parameters are controlled.

If the bathing medium is of a different temperature or pH to that of the former lens storage medium, then time must be allowed for the radius of the lens to stabilize. In this situation, the practitioner should continue to take measurements over a period of several minutes until the radius measurement stabilizes. Keeping the lens in the solution for several minutes before measuring its radius will also allow the lens to revert to its original shape after being distorted during removal from its storage vial (Chaston and Fatt, 1980). Currently, the Optimec instrument is the only one of the three instruments mentioned that is available with a temperature control for the saline bath.

Measurement of the sag of a lens with ultrasound

Port (1979) has described a technique for measuring the sag of a lens with an ultrasonic beam. The design produced by Port shows the contact lens supported on a solid cylinder of known diameter in a bath of saline (*see Figure 11.16*). An ultrasonic transducer is also placed in the bath which sends an ultrasonic beam towards the lens and receives the beam reflections from the lens surfaces and lens support. These reflections are then displayed on an oscilloscope as shown in *Figure 11.16*(b). From a knowledge of the velocity of sound in saline, the time interval between the reflections from the back of the lens and its support can be converted into a linear distance. Port (1979) claims that the accuracy of the ultrasonic technique is of the order of 0.05 mm of radius when it is used on a series of known hard radii. In practice, it is difficult to obtain a true measure of its accuracy on hydrophilic lenses because no standard hydrophilic lenses exist. It can be assumed, however, that once the lens has stabilized the accuracy of a measurement will be very close to that mentioned above for hard surfaces.

A commercially available ultrasonic sag measuring device is manufactured by Panametrics (US) and marketed in the UK by Focus Contact Lenses. In this instrument, the oscilloscope is replaced by an electronic circuit which converts the signal into a measurement of sag, which is then digitially displayed. As with the Kelvin soft lens measuring gauge, the Panametrics ultrasonic radiusope does not incorporate any means of either

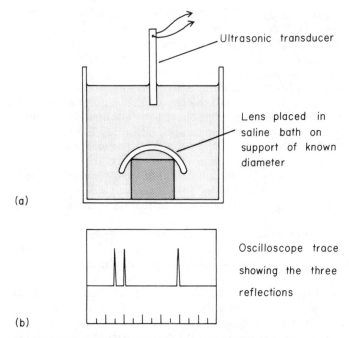

Ultrasonic transducer

Lens placed in saline bath on support of known diameter

(a)

Oscilloscope trace showing the three reflections

(b)

Figure 11.16. (a) Apparatus for the measurement of the sag with ultrasound. (b) Oscilloscope trace showing the reflections from the lens surface and support. After Port (1979)

measuring or controlling the temperature or tonicity of the bathing medium. Chaston and Fatt (1980) report that it is occasionally difficult to obtain a measurement with this instrument from lenses with high water content. The difficulty is due to the strength of reflections decreasing as the acoustic index of the lens approaches that of the bathing medium

While, in theory, the ultrasonic technique can also be used to measure the central thickness of contact lenses, it requires a knowledge of the velocity of sound in each type of lens material. This information is not readily available.

Measurement of the sag from a projected profile

The sag of a lens can be measured from its projected profile. Kawabe and Hamano (1977) have described a technique whereby a projection microscope is used to produce a projected profile of a lens which is supported in a saline cell. Orthogonal scales on the screen are used to obtain a measure of the sag, the centre thickness and the overall size of the lens.

Drysdale's principle of measuring the radii of curvature

At the turn of the century, Drysdale developed a technique to measure the radius of curvature of surfaces of short radius, such as microscope objectives. His technique has been adopted by the optometric profession in order to measure the radii of curvature of contact lenses.

Drysdale's technique requires a compound microscope in which a target is projected along the axis of the instrument (*see Figure 11.17*(a)). An image of this target will be seen through the microscope when it is focused upon a reflecting surface, such as a contact lens. An image will also be seen when the microscope is focused at the centre of curvature of a concave or convex surface due to the light being reflected back along its path by the curved surface (*see Figure 11.17*(a) and (b)). The distance between the two positions, where an in-focus image of the target is seen, equals the radius of

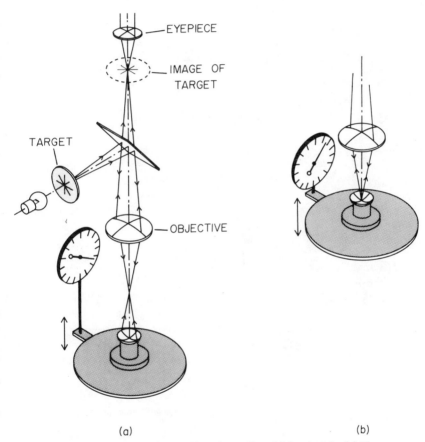

(a)   (b)

Figure 11.17. The optics of a radiuscope based upon Drysdale's principle. (a) The microscope is focused at the radius of curvature of the lens. (b) It is focused on the surface of the lens

curvature of that surface. By attaching a measuring device, such as a dial gauge, to the side of the microscope, a measurement of this distance can be obtained. Radiuscopes based upon Drysdale's principles are made by several instrument manufacturers, including American Optical, Kelvin (*see Figure 11.18*), Neitz, Nissel and Topcon. They differ only in mechanical details.

Hard contact lenses are normally floated on a small pool of water during the measurement of their radii in order to reduce the reflections from the surface not being measured. Care must be taken when floating the lens in this way not to knock the instrument during the measurement process as this can result in a slight movement of the lens and a consequent error in the measured radius. Even with this problem, the accuracy of the technique is of a high order. Loran and French (1978) give the standard deviation of a series of 25 measurements with the American Optical radiuscope as being 0.03 mm.

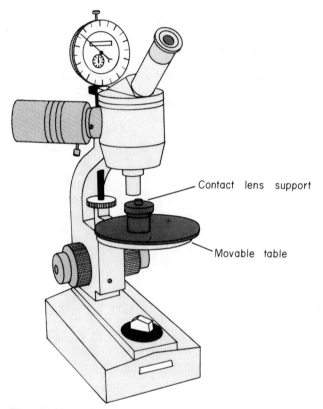

Contact lens support

Movable table

Figure 11.18. The Kelvin monocular radiuscope

Radiuscopes based upon Drysdale's technique can be used to measure the peripheral radii of hard contact lenses by inclining the lens during the measurement process. While, in theory, a measurement can be made over a very small region of the lens, in practice it is difficult to measure peripheral curves which are less than 0.2 mm in width. This is partially due to the difficulty in positioning the lens with sufficient accuracy. A big advantage of Drysdale's radiuscope over many of the other radius measuring devices is that it can be used to measure toric surfaces. Its target is designed to be sensitive to toric surfaces and to allow easy measurement of the radius along each of the meridians.

Drysdale's radiuscope can, with the aid of a special wet cell, also be used to measure the radii of soft contact lenses (*see Figure 11.19*). The wet cell contains saline at some predetermined temperature and tonicity. Rogers (1979) recommends 20 °C (room temperature) and a tonicity of 0.9 per cent saline, which is equivalent to that of most storage solutions used by manufacturers when they dispatch lenses. The transparent lid placed on the top of the cell eliminates the saline–air interface, which would otherwise reduce the quality of the mire image. Because the lens is immersed in saline, the radiuscope reading has to be multiplied by the refractive index of saline (1.336) in order to obtain a measurement of the contact lens radius.

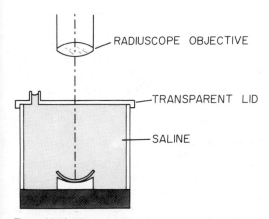

RADIUSCOPE OBJECTIVE

TRANSPARENT LID

SALINE

Figure 11.19. The wet cell used to measure the radius of curvature of soft contact lenses with a radiuscope based upon Drysdale's principle. After Chaston (1978)

There are two problems that arise from using the wet cell. First, the mire image is very faint due to the relatively small amount of light being reflected from the saline–lens interface. This problem has been overcome with the development of an instrument called the Ultra Radiuscope which is made by Canoptica Laboratory, Madrid. This instrument has a very powerful fan-cooled light source which produces a much brighter mire image. In addition to this, it differs from a conventional radiuscope in that the objective of the microscope is immersed in the saline with the contact lens, thereby eliminating the need for a transparent lid on the top of the wet cell.

The second problem is that two sets of reflections of approximately equal brightness occur from the lens: one set from the front surface and one from the back. Chaston (1978) claims that differentiation between these reflections is not difficult. The bottom two reflections, those that occur when the microscope is focused on the surfaces of the lens, can be distinguished by their relative position, the lower one being from the front surface. The top two can be distinguished from a knowledge of the lens power. If the lens is positively powered, then the first reflection encountered as the microscope is racked up will be from the front surface. If it is negatively powered, then it will be from the back surface.

TABLE 11.1. The accuracy of several instruments in the measurement of soft lens radii. (After Loran and French, 1978)

Instrument	Sample statistics (n = 25)	
	SD	*Range*
Ultra Radiuscope	0.023	0.10
Zeiss (Oberkochen) Ophthalmometer	0.051	0.26
Söhnges Projection System	0.076	0.30
Contact Lens Manufacturing Wet Cell Gauge	0.096	0.35
Wöhlk Microspherometer	0.170	0.60
American Optical Radiuscope (using a hard lens)	0.030	0.26

Loran and French (1978) have evaluated the accuracy of the Ultra Radiuscope. They measured the same soft lens 25 times and found the standard deviation of the measurments to be 0.023 mm. They repeated the experiment with five other radius measuring devices and found that none of them gave as good a result as the Ultra Radiuscope (*see Table 11.1*).

Measurement of the radius by comparison with templates

One of the simplest means of checking the radii of soft contact lenses is with a series of acrylic spheres of known radii of curvature (*see Figure 11.20*)*. The base curve of the contact lens is found by transferring it from sphere to sphere until an alignment between the lens and a sphere is obtained. Alignment is recognized by the absence of a bubble at either the centre or edge of the lens.

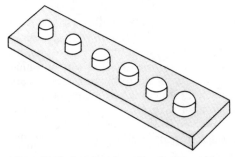

Figure 11.20. A series of acrylic spheres used to check the radius of curvature of soft contact lenses

The spheres are usually made in 0.3 mm steps which means that the technique can only give a rough guide as to the base curve of the lens. Harris, Hall and Oye (1973) produced a series of spheres with 0.1 mm steps, but found it impossible to distinguish differences in base curves of less than 0.3 mm.

* A set of such spheres can be obtained from most contact lens prescription houses

The Hydro-Vue soft lens analyzer utilizes this technique. The posts are, however, submerged in saline and the judgement of alignment is made by viewing the projected profile of the lens and post rather than by looking for bubbles. The posts of the Hydro-Vue instrument are made in 0.2 mm steps. Interpolation between posts will therefore give a base curve reading to the nearest 0.1 mm. Chaston and Fatt (1980) point out that the lens may become distorted when transferred from one post to another, with the result that it may take several minutes before it reverts to its original shape. The instrument has been reviewed by Davis and Anderson (1979) who found that with 10 duplicate measurements, two gave a different value for the base curve.

The Söhnges Kontr-mess instrument projects a profile of the lens, which is contained within a wet cell, onto a screen positioned approximately 1 m from the projector (Söhnges, 1974). Engraved upon the screen are a series of annuli graduated in 0.1 mm steps from 7.20 to 9.50 mm of radius. These can be adjusted vertically and compared with the projected profile of the lens. Loran (1974) has evaluated the instrument and claims that the radius can easily be measured to an accuracy of 0.1 mm and, with practice, to 0.05 mm by interpolation. Linear scales on the screen also allow the practitioner to measure the overall size of the lens and its thickness. Being able to measure more than one parameter with the same instrument is a big advantage in a busy practice, especially when one considers that the practitioner may have to wait a minute or two after a lens has been placed within a wet cell in order for its parameters to settle down to a stable value. The Hydro-Marc Comparator and Marco Lens Comparator operate on similar principles, but are more compact than the Söhnges instrument.

Lens thickness measuring devices

The thickness of spectacle lenses and contact lenses can be measured with the following instruments and techniques:

1. Thickness measuring gauge (spectacle lenses and hard contact lenses);
2. A modified micrometer (soft contact lenses only);
3. Drysdale's radiuscope (spectacle lenses, hard contact lenses and soft contact lenses);
4. By measurement from a projected profile (hard and soft contact lenses) (*see* Söhnges instrument above and Optimec instrument, pp. 220–221);
5. With Ultrasonography (hard and soft contact lenses), *see* pp. 221–222.

Thickness measuring gauge

The thickness of spectacle lenses and all types of hard contact lenses can be measured with this instrument (*see Figure 11.21*). The dial is normally calibrated with a 0.01 mm scale. Care must be taken when using this gauge to ensure that the lens surface is normal to the plunger or else a thicker

228

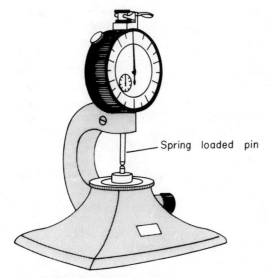

Figure 11.21. The thickness gauge

than true reading will be obtained. The practitioner can verify that the lens is normal to the posts by viewing the dial while gently rocking the lens. The minimum reading will occur when the posts are normal to the lens surface.

A modified micrometer

Fatt (1977) described a technique for measuring the thickness of soft contact lenses with a modified engineer's micrometer. The instrument, which is shown in *Figure 11.22*, relies upon the electrical conductivity of soft lenses. A special lens support, which contains an electrode, is placed over the bottom post of the micrometer. This electrode and a wire from the

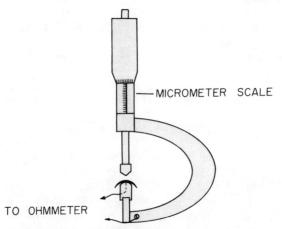

Figure 11.22 A modified micrometer used to measure the thickness of soft contact lenses. After Fatt (1977)

body of the micrometer are connected to an ohmmeter. With the contact lens placed on the lens support, the upper post is gradually screwed down until the ohmmeter reading is seen to drop suddenly. A reading from the micrometer is then taken, which, when subtracted from the base line reading (the same procedure only with the lens removed), will give a measure of the soft lens thickness.

The technique has been evaluated by Pearson (1980b) who found it to have a lower standard deviation of results than all the techniques which use Drysdale's radiuscope. He did, however, find it impossible to get a consistent result from ultra thin lenses and suggested that the variability was due to the varying thickness of the surface water film.

Fatt's design has been incorporated in the Rehder ST-2 sagittal height and thickness gauge (Pollock, 1981).

Measurement of contact lens thickness with a Drysdale radiuscope

The radiuscope can be used to measure the *thickness* of a contact lens (hard or soft). There are three ways in which this can be done:

1. By measuring the real thickness in air;
2. By measuring the apparent thickness in air;
3. By measuring the apparent thickness in saline.

By measuring the real thickness in air

The microscope is first of all focused upon its stage and then, after the lens has been placed on the stage (convex side down), refocused on the lens' back surface. The distance that the microscope has been racked up will equal the thickness of the contact lens.

By measuring the apparent thickness in air

With the lens in place on the stage, the microscope is first of all focused on the lens' front surface and then on the lens' back surface. The distance that the microscope has moved will equal the apparent thickness of the lens which can be converted into the true thickness by multiplying by the refractive index of the lens material.

By measuring the apparent thickness in saline

This technique is the same as the measurement in air, with the exception that the lens is placed within a wet cell.

Pearson (1980b) has evaluated all three techniques and concludes that they all give a similar degree of accuracy. Standard deviations were found to range from 0.006 to 0.013 mm and were generally larger on soft lenses. He found it impossible to obtain a measure of the thickness on an ultra thin lens (centre thickness 0.06 mm) and on a high water content lens with the final technique because of an inability to obtain an image from the back surface of the lens.

References

BENNETT, A. G. (1968). *Emsley and Swaine's Ophthalmic Lenses,* Vol. 1. Hatton Press, London

CHASTON, J. (1978). The verification of the optical dimensions of the soft lens. In *Soft Contact Lenses: Clinical and Applied Technology,* p. 457. Edited by M. Ruben. Balliere Tindall, London

CHASTON, J. and FATT, I. (1980). Survey of commercially available instruments for measuring back radius of soft contact lenses. *Optician,* **179,** May 2nd, 19

DAVIS, H. E. and ANDERSON, D. J. (1979). An investigation of the reliability of hydrogel lens parameters. *International Contact Lens Clinic,* **6,** 136

FATT, I. (1977). A simple electric device for measuring thickness and sagittal height of gel lenses. *Optician,* **173,** March 4th, 23

HAMANO, H. and KAWABE, H. (1978). Method of measuring radii of a soft lens with an electronic device. *Contacto,* **22,** 4

HARRIS, M. G., HALL, K. and OYE, R. (1973). The measurement and stability of hydrophilic lens dimensions. *American Journal of Optometry and Physiological Optics,* **50,** 546

KAWABE, H. and HAMANO, H. (1977). Standardisation of soft contact lenses (second report). *Contacto,* **21,** 15

LORAN, D. F. C. (1974). Determination of hydrogel contact lens radii by projection. *Ophthalmic Optician,* **14,** 980

LORAN, D. F. C. and FRENCH, C. N. (1978). The efficacy of verifying the base curve of hydrogel contact lenses. *International Contact Lens Clinic,* **5,** 39

PEARSON, R. M. (1980a). Wet cell measurement of soft lens power. *Journal of the British Contact Lens Association,* **3,** 13

PEARSON, R. M. (1980b). Measurement of centre thickness of soft lenses. *Contacto,* **24,** 9

POLLOCK, S. L. (1981). A contact lens sagittal height and thickness gauge. *American Journal of Optometry and Physiological Optics,* **58,** 640

PORT, M. (1979). The measurement of soft lens surfaces using ultrasound. *Contacto,* **23,** 5

PORT, M. (1980). The radius measurement of soft lenses in air. *Journal of British Contact Lens Association,* **3,** 168

PORT, M. (1981). The Optimec contact lens analyser. *Optician,* **181,** April 3rd, 11

POSTER, M. G. (1971). Hydrated method of determining dioptral power of a hydrophilic lens. *Journal of American Optometry Association,* **42,** 369

POSTER, M. G. and SKOLNIK, A. J. (1974). Effect of pH and tonicity changes on some parameters of Soflens (TM). *Journal of the American Optometry Association,* **45,** 311

ROGERS, J. E. (1979). Instrumentation used in contact lens verification, 1. *Optician,* **177,** May 25th, 25

SARVER, M. D. and KERR, K. (1964). A radius of curvature measuring device for contact lenses. *American Journal of Optometry and Archives of American Academy of Optometry,* **41,** 481

SARVER, M. D., HARRIS, M. G., MANDELL, R. B. and WEISSMAN, B. A. (1973). Power of Bausch and Lomb Soflens contact lenses. *American Journal of Optometry and Physiological Optics,* **50,** 195

SÖHNGES, C. P. (1974). A Söhnges control and measuring unit for hard and soft contact lenses. *Contacto,* **18,** 31

WICHTERLE, O. (1965). Les lentilles de contact souples 'Getakt': Problemes techniques et chimiques. *Les Cahiers des Verres de Contact,* **6,** 4

WOODCOCK, F. R. (1980). Projection focimeters. *Manufacturing Optics International,* **33(6),** 19

12

Screeners

Introduction

There are many visual conditions that can create a decrement in visual performance and yet which do not yield a set of symptoms that would automatically result in the patient seeking professional advice. One of the most obvious situations where this occurs is in young children. The failure of a child to see clearly can affect his progress in school and yet need not result in any complaint from the child. Screening programmes are designed to avoid the occurrence of such situations. Patients are examined within a screening programme irrespective of whether they have any known visual disability.

Screening programmes are normally carried out by either governmental organizations, such as education authorities, or by employers. The employers include such programmes either as part of a general welfare programme for their employees or in order to check that their employees can efficiently perform a certain visual task while at work.

The number and type of tests carried out within a screening programme varies with the screening authority. Some authorities may be content to know that those tested have a reasonably good distance acuity, while others may want all of those tested to undergo a full eye examination including a refraction. Generally, most authorities are interested in establishing that those tested have good acuity (distance and near), good stereopsis and normal colour vision. In order to meet the requirements of these authorities, certain instrument manufacturers have designed equipment that is capable of measuring these basic functions. These instrumental vision screeners are attractive to many screening authorities as they give a simple pass or fail result and do not require any professional judgements to be made. Those failing the test are simply referred to an optometrist for further examination.

In the remainder of this chapter, I describe these instruments and the types of test they incorporate. At the very end of the chapter, I briefly describe some of the criticisms levelled at the instruments.

Instrumental vision screeners

Practically all visual screening instruments are based upon the Brewster
–Holmes stereoscope. This stereoscope, which is shown in *Figure 12.1*,
utilizes decentred +5.00 D lenses in order to dissociate the two eyes.
Specially designed cards, placed within the card holder of the stereoscope,
can simultaneously present either the same image to each eye or totally
different images. The amount of accommodation required to see these
clearly is dependent upon the distance of the card holder from the lenses.
When it is 20 cm from the lenses, the patient has to exert zero accommodation. The amount of convergence necessary to fuse similar targets is
dependent upon the amount of target separation.

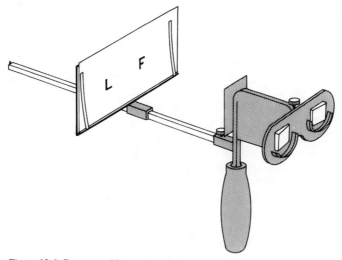

Figure 12.1. Brewster–Holmes stereoscope

Instrumental vision screeners are, in essence, a Brewster–Holmes
stereoscope with a series of different cards. Each card tests one of the basic
visual functions, such as acuity and stereopsis. They may, to allow
convenient presentation, be mounted on a drum or wheel and be completely enclosed within the instrument (*see Figure 12.2*). Because many of the
tests are sensitive to the type and standard of illumination, most screening
instruments incorporate their own illumination systems.

While some instruments have only a single set of cards that are designed
to give either a general screening or a screening for a specific visual task
(such as driving), other instruments, e.g. the Keystone Ophthalmic
Telebinocular, allow the types of cards used within the instrument to be
altered. The manufacturers of these instruments invariably offer several
series of cards each of which is designed to test for a specific type of task.
They also allow the screening authority to devise their own series of cards.

The criterion for passing the tests incorporated within a given visual
screener is set by the screening authority, although guidelines are usually
provided by the manufacturers. By changing the passing criterion of

individual tests, the authorities can match the visual capabilities of those tested with the foreseen visual requirements. For instance, if a screening instrument was used by a company who believed that good distance acuity was important, they could set the screener to fail patients who did not have an equivalent Snellen acuity of 6/5. If, on the other hand, the screener was

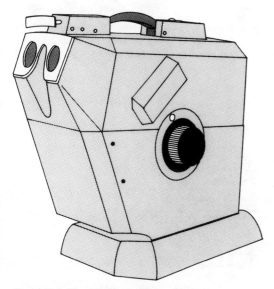

Figure 12.2. Fleming Master Vision Screener, Mavis (British American Optical)

being used by a company employing clerical workers who needed good near acuities, they could set the instrument to fail patients not capable of reading N5 type.

The types of tests normally included in instrumental vision screeners

Visual acuity

Visual acuity is usually measured at both distance and near. The instrument may use conventional letter charts, such as illiterate Es, or it may use specially designed optotypes, such as those shown in *Figure 12.3*. While the Goldmann and Orthorater optotypes measure the resolving power of the eye, the Keystone acuity test measures detectability. While detectability is related to resolving power, it is not the same thing.

Bailey (1973) has compared Snellen acuity measurements with those obtained from eight different vision screeners. In general terms he found that all of the instruments, with the exception of the Orthoscope, gave acceptably valid measures of the distance acuity, only rarely differing by the equivalent of one Snellen line. The Orthoscope, which uses Landolt Cs for the measurement of distance acuity, was occasionally found in error by

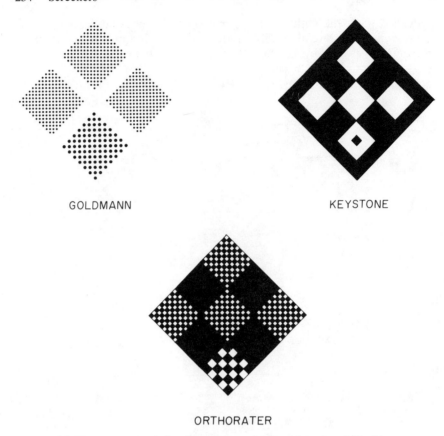

GOLDMANN   KEYSTONE

ORTHORATER

Figure 12.3. Three optotypes designed for the measurement of visual acuity in vision
screeners. With the Goldmann and Orthorater optotypes the patient has to report the
position of the coarse dots or chequered pattern; with the Keystone optotype the
patient has to report the position of the small square

more than one Snellen line. Bailey (1973) points out that most screening
instruments have a relatively small number of optotypes at each acuity step
and that, while this speeds up the process of measuring the acuity, it leads
to a greater scatter of results.

Colour vision

Several screeners incorporate a series of isochromatic charts in order to
assess whether the patients have defective colour vision. The number of
charts included in any one instrument is far below that found in a standard
set of isochromatic plates and thus the sensitivity of this test is low. As the
commercially available sets of isochromatic plates are themselves designed
to screen colour vision and do not require a professional to administer
them, it would seem much wiser for those persons who require a colour
vision test to screen separately with a set of isochromatic plates.

Stereopsis

Most instruments incorporate a test of stereopsis in which one of a series of targets presented to each eye is seen with a small retinal disparity. The patient has to report which target appears to stand out, i.e. which has the disparity. With a series of such tests, each with a different sized disparity, the approximate stereo-acuity of the patient can be measured. Stereopsis tests of this kind are particularly good at revealing binocular problems, although a disadvantage of incorporating them in a screening instrument is that failure of the stereopsis test does not necessarily mean that the patient has poor stereopsis: it may merely indicate an uncorrected refractive error.

Heterophoria

The majority of visual screening instruments incorporate a test that measures the patient's heterophoria. The test is usually based upon a dissociation technique. One of the problems encountered with measuring the distance heterophoria is that the known proximity of the target often stimulates the eye to converge. This phenomena is known as proximal convergence and its effect is to produce a larger measure of distance esophoria (or reduced measure of distance exophoria) than truly exists.

Fogging tests

In order to screen out hyperopic patients, several of the vision screeners incorporate either a +1.00 D (Rodatest R7) or +2.00 D (Fleming Master Vision Screener) fogging test. Hyperopic patients will not be fogged by these lenses to the same extent as normal patients.

Suppression

Two of the instruments listed in *Table 12.1* contain a test of suppression. However, this test is really superfluous if stereopsis has already been measured.

A summary of the tests incorporated in many of the currently produced vision screeners is given in *Table 12.1*. As can be seen, the Keystone instrument offers by far the widest range of tests.

The value of instrumental vision screeners

One of the ways of evaluating a vision screener is to measure the number of over and under referrals that it produces. Over referrals are those cases where the patient fails the test, but is subsequently found to have nothing wrong with vision. Under referrals are cases where patients pass the screening test, but do, in fact, have a visual defect. Generally, instrumental vision screeners fail about 30 per cent of tested patients. On further examination, many of these are found to be over referrals, possibly produced by a lack of understanding by the patient as to what exactly he or

TABLE 12.1. A summary of the tests incorporated in many of the currently manufactured vision screeners

	Fleming Master Vision Screener (Mavis) BAO	Titmus Vision Screener[a]	Ophthalmic Telebinocular Keystone[b,c]	Topcon Screenoscope Tokyo	Rodatest R9 Rodenstock[a]	Rodatest R7 Rodenstock	Sight Screener AO	Master Orthorator Bausch and Lomb[e]
Total no. targets	14	12	15	16	9	10	14	12
No. distant targets	7	6	9	8	5	5	7	7
No. near targets	7{6(33 cm), 1(20 cm)}	6	6(any dist.)	8(30 cm)	4{1(33 cm), 3(25 cm)}	5(28 cm)	7(33 cm)	5(33 cm)
Acuity type	Series of words	Landolt Cs	Snellen	Illiterate Es	Chequerboard	Goldmann	Snellen	Chequerboard
Colour vision	–	Pseudo-isochromatic	Pseudo-isochromatic	–	–	–	Colour naming	Pseudo-isochromatic
Stereopsis	Dist. + Nr.	–	Dist.	Dist. + Nr.	Dist.	Dist. + Nr.	Dist. + Nr.	Dist.
Heterophoria[f] distant	V + H	V + H	V + H	H	V + H	V + H	V + H	V + H
near	V + H	V + H	V + H	H	V + H	V + H	V + H	V + H
Fogging test	+ 2.00 D	–	–	–	–	+1.00 D	–	–
Suppression	–	–	Fusion	–	–	–	Dist. + Nr.	–

a   Can get a different series of charts for aviation testing
b   Keystone also manufacture a screener designed to test drivers
c   Offers the largest range of cards (up to 29) which can be used in any sequence
d   Rodenstock also manufacture two other screeners, the R5 and R3. The R5 is specially designed for children and the R3 for drivers.
e   A modified version is available with different types of acuity charts
f   V = vertical; H = horizontal.

she was supposed to do. In a study on school children, Peters *et al.* (1959) found that when a careful examination was carried out by an optometrist about 18 per cent of children were found to have a visual defect (i.e. nearly half the number of referrals made by instrumental vision screeners). Peters *et al.* (1959) maintain that because of the high referral rate of instrumental screeners and the subsequent demand upon the time of optometrists, it is, in fact, cheaper to use an optometrist to quickly examine all the patients rather than to use an instrumental screener. Peters *et al.* (1959) also found that a modified clinical routine performed by optometrists resulted in a lower under referral rate when compared with instrumental vision screeners.

References

BAILEY, I. L. (1973). Vision screening in industry: Objectives and methods. *Australian Journal of Optometry*, **56,** 70

PETERS, H. B., BLUM, H. L., BETTMAN, J. W., JOHNSON, F. and FELLOWS, V. (1959). The Orinda study. *American Journal of Optometry and the Archives of the American Academy of Optometry*, **36,** 455

Appendix

Conversion factors for luminance units*

	Footlamberts (ftL)	Millilamberts (mL)	Apostilbs (asb)
1 ftL (or 1 lm/ft^2)	1	1.076	1.076×10
1 mL (or 10 lm/cm^2)	9.29×10^{-1}	1	10
1 asb (or 1 lm/m^2)	9.29×10^{-2}	10^{-1}	1
1 cd/m^2	2.92×10^{-1}	3.14×10^{-1}	3.14

* The International Perimetric Society (IPS) have published a *Perimetric Standards* (publ. W. Junk, The Hague) covering luminance and other aspects of perimetry. This table reproduced, with permission, from Bedwell, *Visual Fields*, Butterworths

Index

239